Milady's
Hair Coloring Techniques

LOUISE COTTER

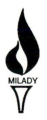

Milady Publishing Company
(A Division of **Delmar Publishers Inc.**)
3 Columbia Circle, Box 15015
Albany, New York 12212-5015

NOTICE TO THE READER

Senior Administrative Editor: Catherine Frangie
Production Manager: John Mickelbank
Developmental Editor: Joe Miranda
Managing Editor: Susan Simpfenderfer
Editorial Production Assistant: Lori McDonald

For information, address Milady Publishing Company
3 Columbia Circle
Albany, New York 12212

COPYRIGHT © 1993
by Milady Publishing Co.
(a division of Delmar Publishers Inc.)

Printed in the United States of America
Published simultaneously in Canada
by Nelson Canada,
a division of The Thomson Corporation

1 2 3 4 5 6 7 8 9 10 XXX 99 98 97 96 95 94 93

Library of Congress Cataloging-in-Publication Data

Cotter, Louise.
    Milady's hair coloring techniques/
    Louise Cotter.
        p. cm.
    ISBN: 1-56253-116-6 (textbook)
    1. Hair — Dyeing and bleaching.   I. Title
TT973.C67 1994
646.7'242 — dc20   92-34185
                                                              CIP

Illustration Credits

Photographers

Chapters 1, 3, 4, 7, 8, 10, 11, 12, 15, 17
Jon Thomas
Jon Thomas Photography
Altamonte Springs, FL

Chapters 5, 9, 13, 14
Norma Lorusso
Lorusso Photography
Charleston, SC

Chapters 2, 6, 16
Beverly Getschel
Bev's Design Studio
Amery, WI

Hair-Color Technicians and Hair Stylists

Chapters 3, 7, 12, 17
Sara Ringler
Sara N'Woody's Beauté Centre
Orlando, FL

Chapters 1, 4, 8
Earline Mallons
Strands Salon
Casselberry, FL

Chapters 10, 11, 15
Chrissy Dunn
Dunn's Beauty Bookings
Orlando, FL

Chapters 2, 6, 16
Beverly Getschel
Bev's Hair Designs
Amery, WI

Chapters 5, 9, 13, 14
Tom Stetser
London Hair Salon
Charleston, SC
Francis London Dubose
Hair Stylist

Makeup Artists

Chapters 3, 7, 12, 17
Sara Ringler, Orlando, FL

Chapters 1, 4, 8
Erline Mallons, Casselberry, FL

Chapters 10, 11, 15
Chrissy Dunn, Orlando, FL

Chapters 2, 6
Laura Wulff, Amery, WI

Chapter 16
Mari Gallogly, St. Paul, MN

Chapters 5, 9, 13, 14
Jennifer Iderton, Charleston, SC

About the Author

LOUISE COTTER is a respected educator and leader in the cosmetology industry. Her dedication to the art of cosmetology is evidenced in her life-long work as a salon owner, instructor, educational director, editor of a major industry magazine, and author of many educational texts.

Ms. Cotter's educational background provided the fundamentals necessary to communicate on multiple levels relating to cosmetology and its many facets. In addition to a wide range of cosmetology skills, her professional expertise extends to art and journalism.

She is a licensed cosmetologist and cosmetology instructor who participates in industry-sponsored events, seminars, and continuing education programs nationwide. She is an accomplished platform artist and lecturer.

Ms. Cotter is a member of the National Cosmetology Association (NCA), NCA Hall of Renown, Michigan Cosmetology Hall of Fame, and the recipient of the first NCA Award of Achievement for excellence in cosmetology education by a cosmetology magazine.

During her 10-year tenure as editor of *American Salon Magazine* she was instrumental in many progressive changes designed to improve the quality of information and education to its readers — some 160,000 salon professionals. *American Salon* is the official publication of the NCA.

As director of education for a chain of cosmetology schools, Ms. Cotter authored much of the supplemental material used in their educational system.

As style director of the NCA's Education and Creative Committee, OHFC/HairAmerica, she was responsible for initiating the first full-size NCA consumer-oriented magazine featuring NCA trends in hair styles, fashion, and positive information promoting professional salon services. After a progression of titles — all meant to epitomize the expertise of NCA's image-making membership — it is now a slick, semiannual publication known as *American Looks*.

Ms. Cotter's contributions to the cosmetology industry and related education are numerous. She participated in the creation of seven NCA Trend Releases, twice served as NCA style director and was a trainer of the 1976 USA Ladies Olympic Hair Styling Team. She is editor and producer of NCA's student membership publication, *FCA Today*.

Education and communication are her mediums. Love of the industry and a sincere wish to perpetuate excellence in cosmetology is her motivation.

Contents

BLEACH AND TONER — ONE COLOR
Original color – Level 7 (warm)
Finished color – Level 10 (palest blonde)
Recommended style: Any style with a smooth to
    moderately layered surface.

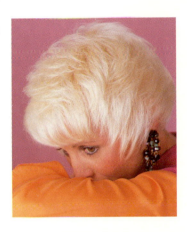

HIGH-LIFT TINT — ONE COLOR
Original color – Level 6 (warm)
Finished color – Level 8 (medium gold-blonde)
Recommended style: Medium blonde colors are
    adaptable to most hair styles – long or short,
    curled or straight.

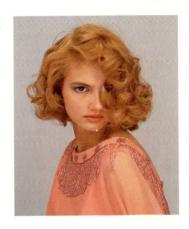

HIGH-LIFT BLEACH AND DARK CONTRAST
Original color – Level 7 (cool)
Finished color – Top: Level 9/10; Bottom: Level 6
Recommended style: Short styles with a definite
    weight line or styles above the ears. Contrast-
    ing colors are best used for accenting a style
    that has a smooth surface with moderate
    movement.

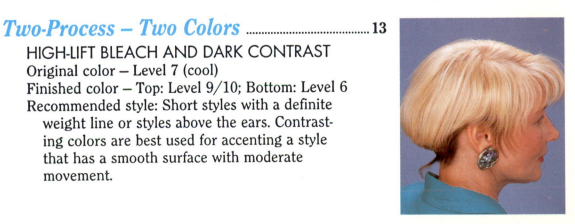

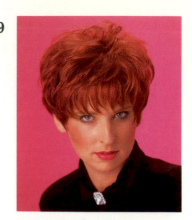
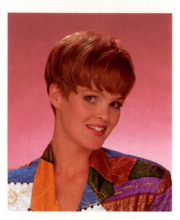
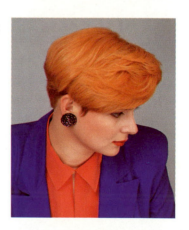
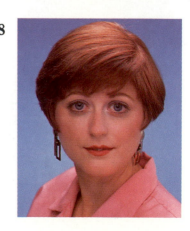

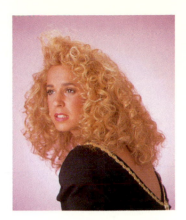

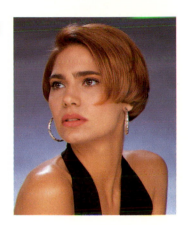

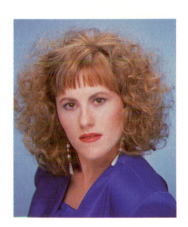

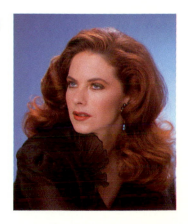

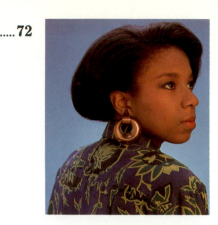

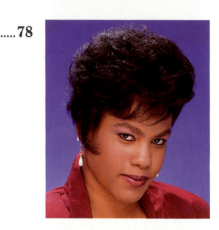

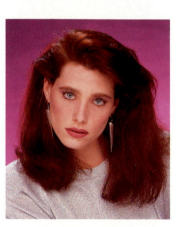

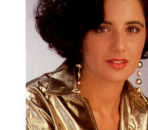

Preface

The purpose of *Hair Coloring Techniques* is to enhance the knowledge of cosmetologists and to supplement material currently available to them. Specifically, it is meant to improve techniques and elevate the technical skills required to execute a variety of color treatments in order to meet the increasing demands of sophisticated consumers.

Most cosmetology courses allot limited classroom hours to the subject of hair color. Practical application is confined to the clinic — and most often to a conservative clientele. Thus, students learn enough hair-color theory to pass a licensing exam. But they lack the expertise and confidence to perform all hair-color services on clients in a full-service salon.

In fact, hair coloring is the weakest skill of most newly licensed cosmetologists — and the most tedious to learn in a salon situation. Working cosmetologists lack the opportunity to experiment. Their only learning experience is at hair-coloring seminars, in private classes, or in salon training.

While education and hands-on experience are major requisites to becoming a skilled colorist, this collection of hair-coloring techniques provides detailed technical information that can easily be followed by the novice or by a seasoned professional.

In order for a student to feel comfortable with color, and as a means of building a trusting color clientele, the application techniques in this book are invaluable. Step-by-step applications along with complete explanations of when, why, and how to master all hair-color possibilities give designers an accelerated course that will make them confident enough to work in the most modern salon.

Being artistic individuals, hair designers and technicians need to stay current and to enjoy the creative possibilities of their profession. This book is conceived and written with that idea in mind.

The rewards of hair-color expertise are many: self-confidence, personal satisfaction, client satisfaction, and unlimited profits for you and your salon.

The concepts in *Hair Coloring Techniques* provide the education necessary to recognize color as an extension of hair design and as an integral part of design composition.

In the ever-changing world of hair styles and fashion apparel, you as a salon professional must know how to recognize the need for style development for your clients. Each trend requires a different approach to exciting color design. It is up to you to suggest color changes and new techniques to accommodate the preferences of the clientele you serve.

Hair Coloring Techniques attempts to hone your skills in those areas. You will learn to understand the technical aspect of color application. Your role as a color technician will become clear, and you can take your place beside the great hair colorists who have contributed their time and expertise to make this collection of hair-coloring techniques the best educational text available.

Louise Cotter
1992

Introduction

WHY SHOULD YOU BE A SKILLED HAIR-COLOR TECHNICIAN?

1. *To satisfy consumer demand*
2. *To increase your income*
3. *To improve your job opportunities*

Hair color is a high-ticket service that accounts for a large percentage of a full-service salon's gross income — a real incentive to perfect the art. Seventy-five percent of adult American females and countless men use some kind of color on their hair. We also know that a high percentage of them use over-the-counter products. The salon professional must be qualified to produce better results than clients can achieve at home in order to gain a greater share of the over-the-counter market.

Hair coloring is not a salon service that can survive poor results. Clients simply will not return to a salon that has botched their hair color. On the other hand, a client will not leave a salon (not even if the designer goes to another salon) if he or she is satisfied with the salon's hair-color service — another reason to increase your knowledge of hair color and improve your technical skills.

America is a youth-oriented society. Physical appearance is increasingly important. Right or wrong, well-groomed, attractive people are perceived to be more capable, better educated and more socially acceptable than those who opt for the natural look.

Only well-trained color technicians are capable of meeting the challenge of constant change in the industry. During the past three decades hair color has been accepted and rejected in cycles. It is widely accepted today because salon professionals elevated their level of expertise while manufacturers refined their products.

Once, it was thought the only reason for coloring one's hair was to cover premature gray. Imitating blonde celebrities was once the primary motivation for women young and old to go "high-blonde."

All salon services lagged somewhat during the back-to-nature movement that invaded American society in the sixties and seventies. It was then that salon professionals discovered a need to sharpen their hair-color expertise and promotional skills. The entire beauty industry recognized that the basis for selling this highly specialized service was *education*.

Today's salon professionals are acutely aware that hair color still does not sell itself — that social attitudes are subject to change. Sophisticated American consumers make decisions and consider all the options. Hair color must be skillfully presented and sold to clients by salon professionals. In order to do this with confidence, they must be skilled in color selection, application, and results.

The appearance of most women and many men would be greatly improved by enhancing or even changing the natural color of their hair. Today's advanced salon technology makes exciting and effective hair colors as easy to obtain as a simple shampoo — colors that not only enhance physical appearance but actually affect people's lives in a positive way.

The hair-color techniques in this book will help you sell a hair color service that's right for each of your clients.

THE KEY TO SUCCESSFUL HAIR COLORING

In order to simplify the art of hair coloring, it is important to review the basic rules of color and familiarize yourself with the universal language and terms related to hair color and hair-color products — and to improve application techniques through information; detailed, illustrated instructions; and *practice*.

While products capable of changing or enhancing natural hair color have been available for decades, only recently has technical comprehension by professionals and the refinement of hair-color products approached perfection — perfection in the sense that more than 75 percent of American women and an increasing number of men not only accept the hair-color concept, but use hair color in some form.

Unfortunately, a high percentage of those who use hair color purchase over-the-counter products and apply it themselves. That simply means professionals working in licensed beauty salons have not garnered a sufficient share of the market.

In a limited survey of women who color their own hair, the reasons given for not going to a professional salon were: at least one bad experience with professional hair coloring; lack of confidence in the salon technician; difficulty in making their wishes clear to the technician; failure of the technician to comply with their wishes, even when clearly understood; and finally — far down the list — high salon prices.

Far too many cosmetologists, even those in full-service salons, do not have a firm grasp of the art of hair-color services in all its forms.

We don't live in a black-and-white world. Nature provides color in elaborate splendor that enhances our lives and is the source of our most creative expression. The skillful use of color is an integral part of paintings, interior decorating, fashion design, landscaping and formal gardens, to name a few examples.

The use of color to decorate the human body can be traced to primitive times. Today women depend on color in the form of skillfully applied makeup and hair color to make personal statements.

The aging of Americans can just as well be called Americans coming of age. Whichever way it is stated, to cosmetology professionals it means that more people are accepting hair color as part of their regular grooming regimen. Personal image is increasingly important. American workplaces are rapidly changing, and the competition for jobs is intensified as they grow scarce. People who want to look younger and better are looking to salon professionals for direction.

This collection of hair-coloring techniques is timely and educational. Hair color is explained beginning with color basics, followed by rules for best results, and finally, seventeen detailed hair-color technicals executed by hair-color experts who are recognized in the industry nationwide.

Color (natural or artificial) is the source of apparent depth, dimension, and reflection of light in any type of hair.

The first and most lasting impression of a hair style is color. Drama and interest is created by the level of color (lightness or darkness), and tone is defined by whether the color is warm (red, orange, or yellow) or cool (blue, violet, or green).

Level

The level of color is also referred to as depth. Almost universally, color depth is measured from values 1 to 10 — 1 is the darkest value, 10 is the lightest.

Levels 1 and 2 encompass the darkest colors (black and darkest brown). Levels 3-7 on the value scale are considered medium shades. Colors between levels 5 and 7 generally contain the reddest pigments. Levels 8, 9, and 10 are the lightest colors.

The value color scale is used to analyze the depth of natural hair colors as well as artificial hair-color products. This value system, more than any other, standardizes color formulas that allow color technicians to perform hair-color services with predictable results.

Tone

The determining factor between the warm and cool classifications is the visible natural hair-color tone. Hair that appears to contain red or yellow strands is considered "warm." Hair containing no red or yellow tones fall into the "cool" tones. Hair-color products with yellow, orange, or red bases are considered warm. Hair-color products with blue, green, or violet bases are considered cool.

The Color Wheel

The color wheel is a valuable tool in learning and executing all hair-color services. Once it is understood that color complements are opposites on the color wheel, it is easy to control the tone and intensity of all colors. Using the color wheel with the value scale is a reliable way to achieve desired tonal quality.

The Many Patterns of Hair-Color Application

The pattern used to apply hair color depends entirely on the desired effect. Before applying hair color in a particular pattern, the following factors must be considered:

1. the length and elevation of the hair on which color will be applied

2. the effect you wish to create

Once those factors are determined, the following general rules may be followed (While creative hair color is not limited to any rigid set of rules, it is wise to consider these guidelines):

If the hair style has a **solid form** (smooth surface) — one color, with identical units, is most suitable.

For a hair style with a **graduated form** (a short nape that gradually lengthens to a visible weight line) — a color progression creates the most dramatic effect.

A hair style that has a **layered form** is most attractive when an alternation of color is applied (two or more colors applied in sequence as highlighting or lowlighting).

Color to Create the Appearance of Texture

Texture is simply whether the surface of a hair style is smooth, wavy, or extra curly. Since nature or chemical restructuring is usually thought to be the source of texture, this text introduces hair coloring as a means to create the illusion of texture.

If the hair is **straight,** the illusion of texture can be created by applying several shades of color to alter light reflection.

If the hair is **wavy,** bold highlights or lowlights must be used in order to be seen in such an abundance of movement.

If the hair is **extra curly,** especially hair that stands away from the head in a regimented form, surface color application has a dramatic effect.

RATIONALE

Hair-Coloring Techniques is presented in an innovative and creative format. Its purpose is to elevate hair coloring, for whatever reason, to a professional level not attainable by laymen or by cosmetologists unskilled in the art of hair color.

The color techniques interpreted throughout this text are clearly illustrated in a step-by-step progression that is easily understood by color specialists and full-service cosmetologists.

Hair-Coloring Techniques combines creative integration of color with logical rationale for both color selection and uncomplicated application.

As intricate and illuminating as the finished colors appear, each application is based on sound color principles — level, tone and intensity.

Principles of Creative Hair-Color Application

A thorough understanding of three rules of hair color is imperative for effective results:

1. the original color, whether chemically treated or virgin hair color
   a. level
   b. tone
   c. intensity

2. the desired color (final result)
   a. level
   b. tone
   c. intensity

3. selection of colors, formulated to produce the precise lift and deposit needed to achieve the desired result

Areas Where Most Color Possibilities Occur

Base area (scalp)

A. A base lighter than the greater mass activates the design interior.

B. A dark base creates the illusion of depth.

C. A base brighter than other integrated colors creates unexpected interest.

Strand area

All strands can be made the same color, or harmonizing colors; or individual strands may be isolated and made lighter or darker, i.e., highlights or lowlights.

Ends (isolated)

Hair ends may be made lighter or darker for special effects or in order to create the illusion of movement within a layered design.

Zone (selected areas)

Placing different colors in selected areas focuses attention and emphasizes creative elements within the hair style.

Two-Process Blonde

BLEACH AND TONER — ONE COLOR

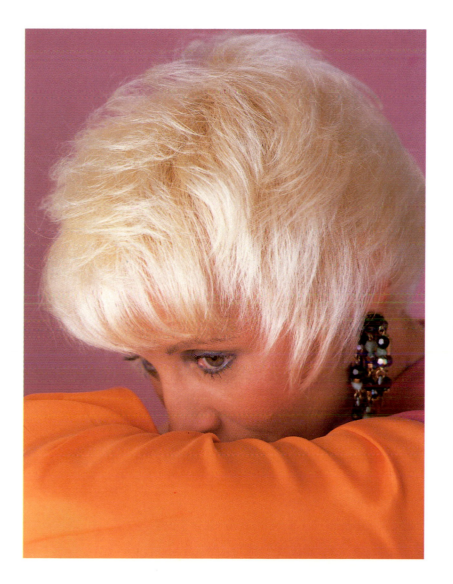

For the client who wants a complete color change and opts for a color several shades lighter than the natural color, the method is almost always a double-process bleach. Many women whose hair is turning gray also prefer to go high-blonde.

To remove natural color from the hair and follow with a toner, the basic rule is to leave only the amount of gold or yellow pigment in the hair that can be covered by the toner.

NO. 1 *Arlene*

ESSENTIALS

COLOR FACTS

The hair can be decolorized to Level 10 (pale yellow). Virgin hair normally goes through ten shades of lightness. The number of levels to be lifted before reaching Level 10 depends on the color level of the natural hair before bleaching. The tonal value of the natural hair — whether it has warm or cool tones — also determines to what degree the hair can be easily bleached.

If the natural hair is Level 7 (medium blonde) with gold (warm) tones, the bleach must remove three levels of natural pigment. Because the hair has gold (warm) tones, some depth of yellow may still remain even after the hair has reached complete decolorization — Level 10. This will determine the selection of toner. A toner with a violet base is most effective for eliminating excessive yellow.

HAIR ANALYSIS

Natural (virgin) hair color — Level 7 (medium blonde); currently 40 percent gray, previously bleached, ½ inch new growth

Tonal value: medium warm

Texture and condition: good

DESIRED COLOR

Warm Iridescent Blonde — Level 10

The client's eye color and skin tone indicate adaptability to pale blonde shades.

FORMULA 1

2 oz. creme bleach

4 oz. 30-volume (9%) peroxide or developer

FORMULA 2

2 oz. pale blonde toner

2 oz. 10-volume (3%) peroxide or developer

SERVICE REQUIRED

Bleach/toner touch-up

PROCEDURE

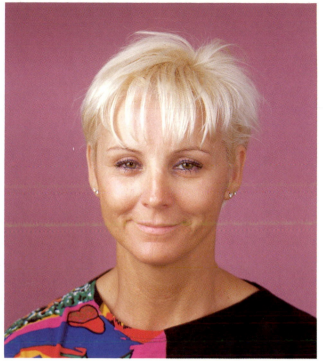

1 The new growth before color application was mousey medium-blonde: color Level 7 with approximately 40 percent gray.

2 Divide the hair into four sections. Make a part from center forehead to center nape and from ear to ear over the crest of the head. Secure each section with long hair clips.

Mix the bleach formula (Formula 1).

Note: The virgin outgrowth is medium-fine and will decolorize quickly. The first application of bleach is applied only at the scalp. Special care is taken not to overlap onto previously bleached strands. The bleach is allowed to remain on the hair only until the scalp area (new growth) has lightened sufficiently.

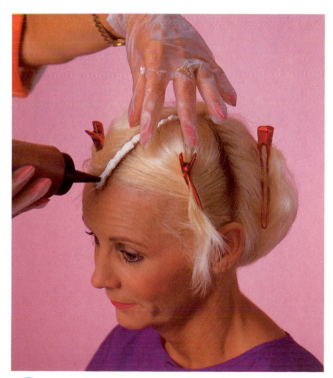

3a Using an applicator bottle, start applying bleach along the part from center forehead to center nape.

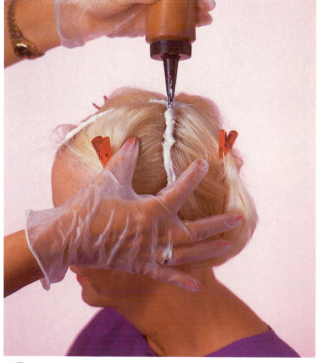

3b Continue applying bleach along the part from ear to ear over the crest of the head.

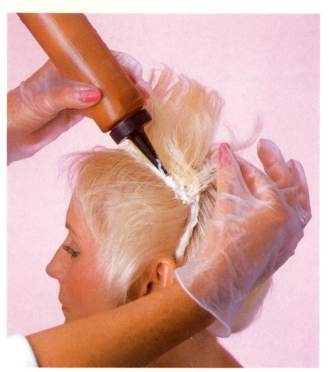

4 Beginning at the top of the left front section, apply bleach to narrow diagonal subsections, working quickly and thoroughly from crown to forehead.

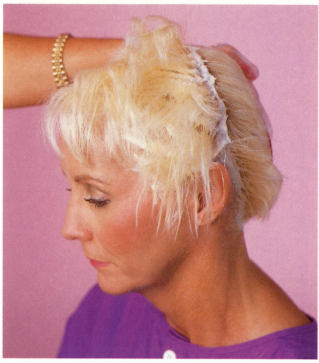

5 When the section is complete, pull the hair strands away from the bleach to avoid contact, and proceed to the three other sections, using the same procedure.

6 Cover the hair loosely to intensify natural body heat at the scalp area, and allow the bleach to process until the scalp area is pale yellow — Level 10.

When desired lift is reached, gently rinse the bleach from the hair with warm, not hot, water. Lightly shampoo the hair (once), without rubbing the scalp, and rinse thoroughly.

7 Towel-dry the hair — do not rub, then dry the hair thoroughly with a hand-held dryer (cool air only). Do not comb or brush the hair any more than necessary to re-section. Divide the hair again into four sections, as in Step 1.

Mix the toner formula (Formula 2) and apply to all the hair at the same time. Allow it to process according to manufacturer's instructions.

Shampoo, rinse, condition if necessary and style the hair.

See finished styles (montage).

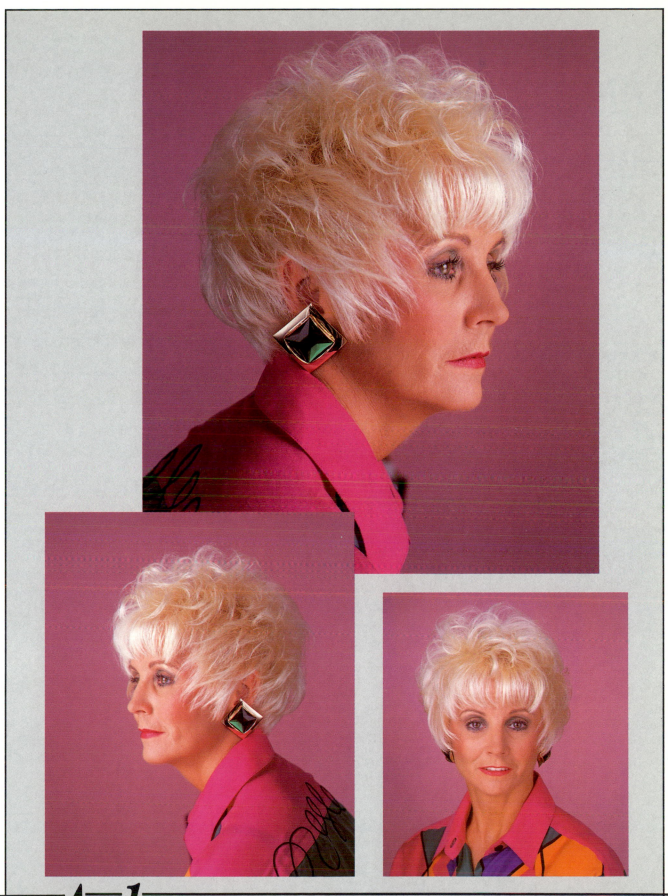

Arlene

One-Process Blonde

HIGH-LIFT TINT — ONE COLOR

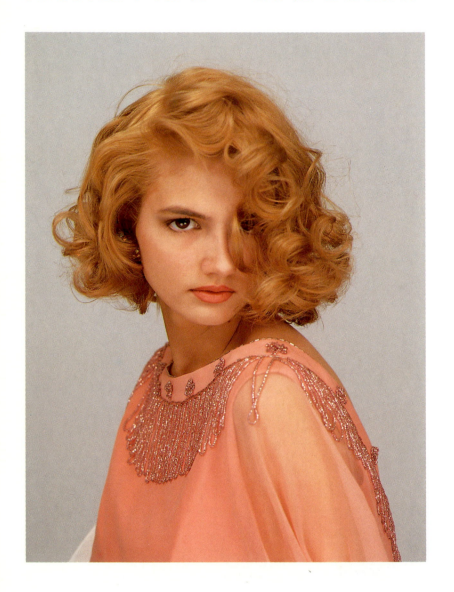

A hair style without layering is considered a solid form. The options for color enhancement or change are many. However, a one-color formula is most attractive on a hair style with a smooth surface.

Color selection for one-color applications is restricted only by the rules governing the amount of lift or deposit that can be attained by the product — and by the natural hair color.

No. **2** *Sharon*

ESSENTIALS

COLOR FACTS

Natural hair color darker than Level 5 can only be lifted to Level 8 by first removing some of the natural pigment (pre-bleaching).

Natural hair within color levels 6-8 has the most options. This natural hair color can be made as light as Level 9 by using a high-lift tint (gold tones will still be in evidence if the tonal value of the natural hair is warm with yellow or red under-tones).

HAIR ANALYSIS

Natural (virgin) hair color — Level 6 (light brown)

Tonal value — medium warm

Porosity — normal

Texture — smooth, close cuticle

DESIRED COLOR

Dark golden blonde — Level 8 (dark golden blonde)

Existing natural color — Level 6 (light brown)

Tonal value — medium warm

Product selection — Liquid tint Level 9

FORMULA 1

2 oz. creme or liquid color — Level 9 (light golden blonde)

2 oz. 30-volume peroxide or developer

1 cap gold concentrate

FORMULA 2

2 oz. creme or liquid color — Level 9 (light golden blonde)

2 oz. 20-volume peroxide or developer

PROCEDURE

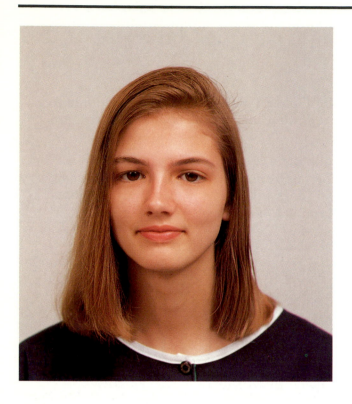

1 The natural hair color as it appeared before color application — drab and without shine

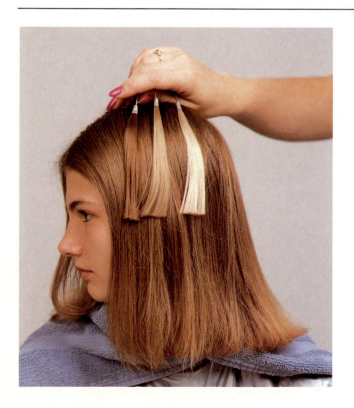

2 Using a professional color ring, isolate three swatches:

1. the closest match to the natural hair color

2. the desired finished color

3. the swatch matching the level of color product applied

This exercise gives you and your client a visual preview of the nearest possible results that can be attained with a one-process procedure. This information provides technical direction and a realistic expectation for the client.

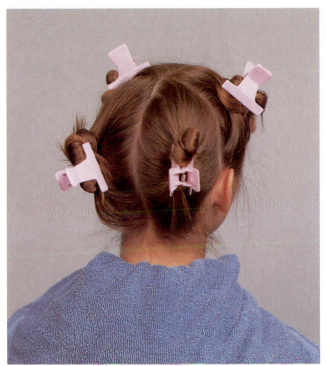

3a Preparation: Divide the hair into four sections. First, make a part from forehead to nape. Secure the section.

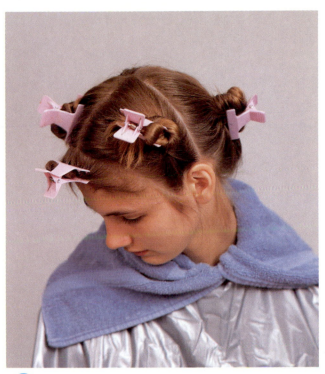

3b Next, make a part from ear to ear over the crest of the head. Secure the section.

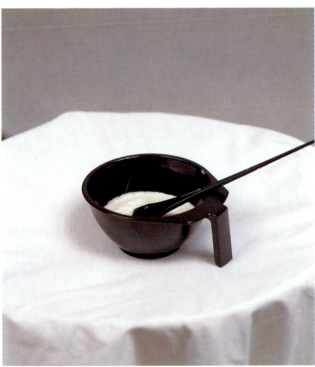

4 Mix batch of Formula 1, using equal amounts of tint and 30-volume peroxide or developer.

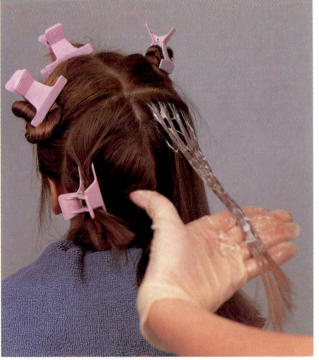

5 Start the fine-brush application at the top of the right back section. Apply formula generously to the hair strand — 1 inch away from the scalp and 1 inch away from the ends.

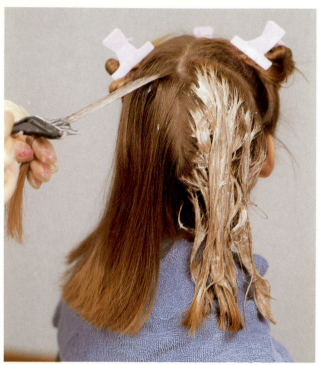

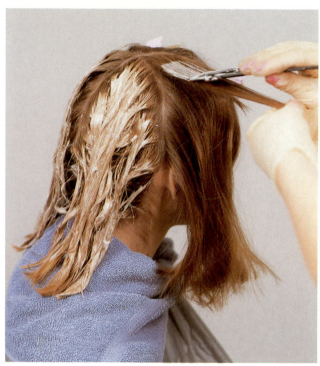

6 Apply formula to the opposite section in the back (1 inch away from the scalp — 1 inch from the ends).

7 Apply Formula 1 to the right front section, using the same procedure used in the back.

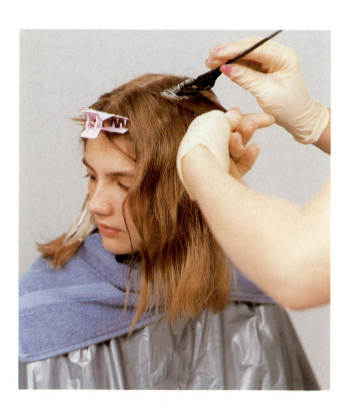

8 Apply Formula 1 to the left front section, using the same method used for the opposite side.

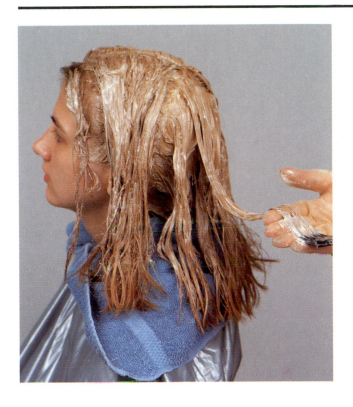

9 Mix batch of Formula 2, using equal amounts of tint and 20-volume peroxide or developer.

Apply Formula 2 to 1-inch area at the scalp and to the ends.

> **Note:** If the ends are excessively porous, reduce the volume of peroxide to 10 or less depending on the degree of porosity.

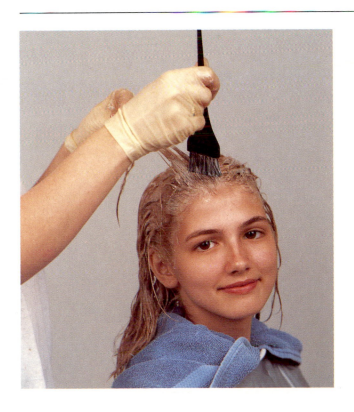

10 Apply Formula 2 to the hairline that frames the face.

Allow the color to process to the desired level. Wash hair; follow with a conditioner only if needed.

See finished styles (montage).

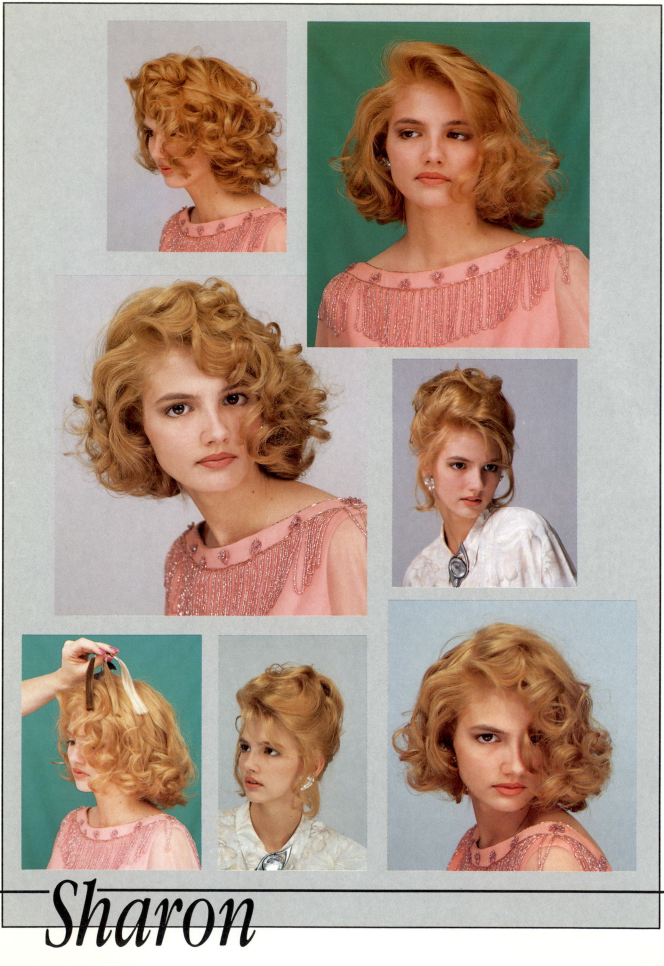

Sharon

Two-Process – Two Colors

HIGH-LIFT BLEACH AND DARK CONTRAST

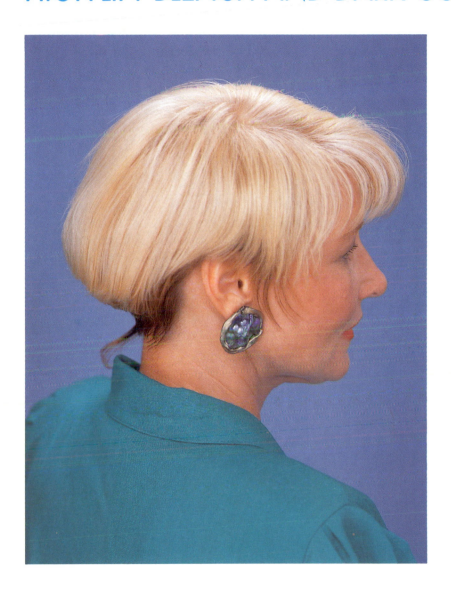

Fashion trends in hair styles often dictate color techniques. When an exaggerated weight line is incorporated into the haircut the style can be enhanced by using light and dark contrasting colors. However if caution and good taste are not exercised in the choice of color, contrasting colors can produce bizarre results. The objective of the two-color technique is to point up the difference between areas. This is far more effective if the difference in the two applied colors is subtle — yet they must be at least three levels apart for the results to be noticeable.

No. **3** *Barbara*

ESSENTIALS

COLOR FACTS

The hair must go through ten levels of decolorizing to reach pale lemon yellow. Levels 7-9 can be achieved with a high-lift tint if the natural hair color is no darker than Level 6.

If the natural hair color is lighter than Level 6, warm blonde levels 8-9 can be achieved without pre-bleaching. If the hair is darker than Level 6 (warm) and the desired color is Level 9 (cool), the hair should be pre-lightened, then toned.

HAIR ANALYSIS

The hair has been previously tinted to Level 7 (dark blonde).

Tonal value — cool

Porosity — excessive

Texture — open cuticle

DESIRED COLOR

It was determined from hair and skin analysis and client consultation that the desired color level is medium warm Level 9. The lower section (nape) and the face frame should be darkened to medium warm Level 6.

FORMULA 1

2 oz. creme or liquid color high-lift tint (lightest golden blonde)

2 oz. 30-volume (9% peroxide or developer)

FORMULA 2

1 oz. creme or liquid color Level 6 (light brown)

1 oz. 10-volume (3% peroxide or developer)

PROCEDURE

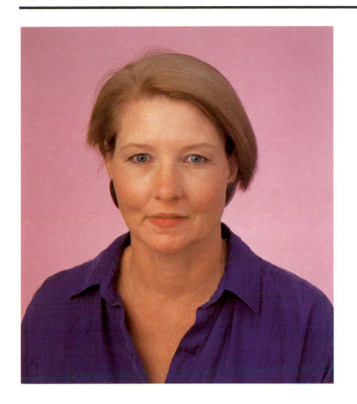

1 The hair, as it appeared before the color change, was drab and damaged.

> **Note:** The hair was re-conditioned two days before color application to equalize porosity.

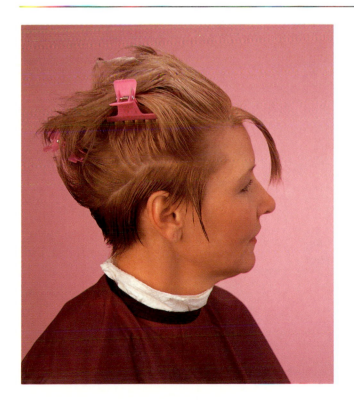

2 Divide the hair in preparation for tinting. Make a part from the forehead to the lower occipital bone (base of skull). Part the hair from ear to ear over the crest of the head, and secure the four crown sections. The area at the nape and a narrow section 1 inch around the face frame and over each ear should be left free.

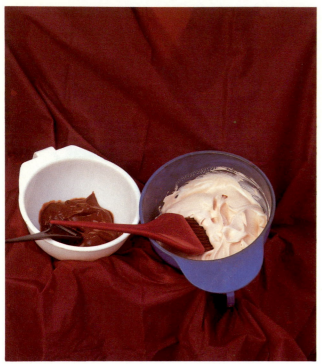

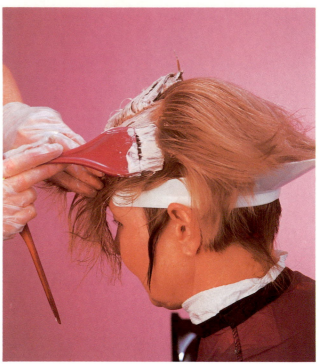

3 Mix two different formulas in separate bowls.

    Formula 1: lighter
    Formula 2: darker

4 Apply Formula 1 to the left front side, avoiding the narrow section that frames the face.

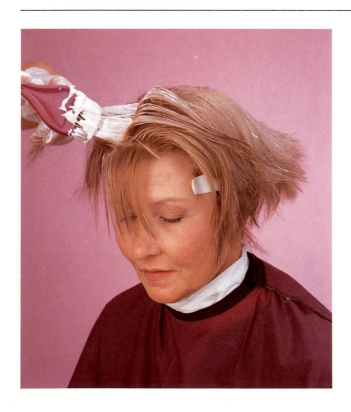

5 Repeat the application with Formula 2 on the right front side, again avoiding the fringe area.

Apply color from scalp to ends to the back sections.

Note: Allow the crown upper section to process for 20 minutes.

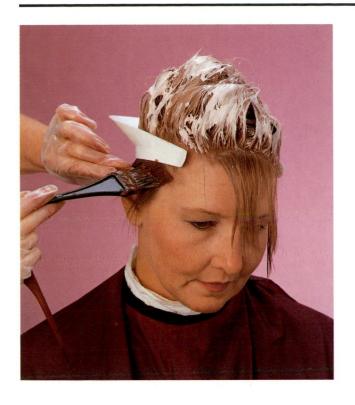

6 Place a plastic shield or aluminum foil from ear to ear at the part separating the nape area from the crown section. This keeps bleach from diluting the tint in the lower section.

Apply formula 2 to the nape area and to the fringe around the face and over the ears.

Allow the entire head to process for another 20 minutes.

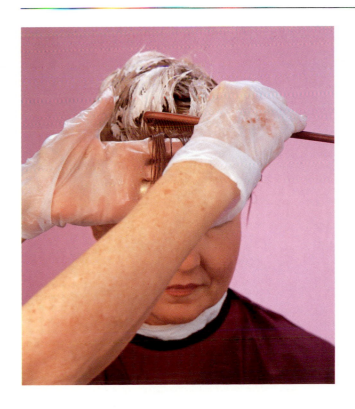

7 Remove the shield and gently blend the two formulas along the part.

Immediately shampoo the hair and condition as necessary.

See finished styles (montage).

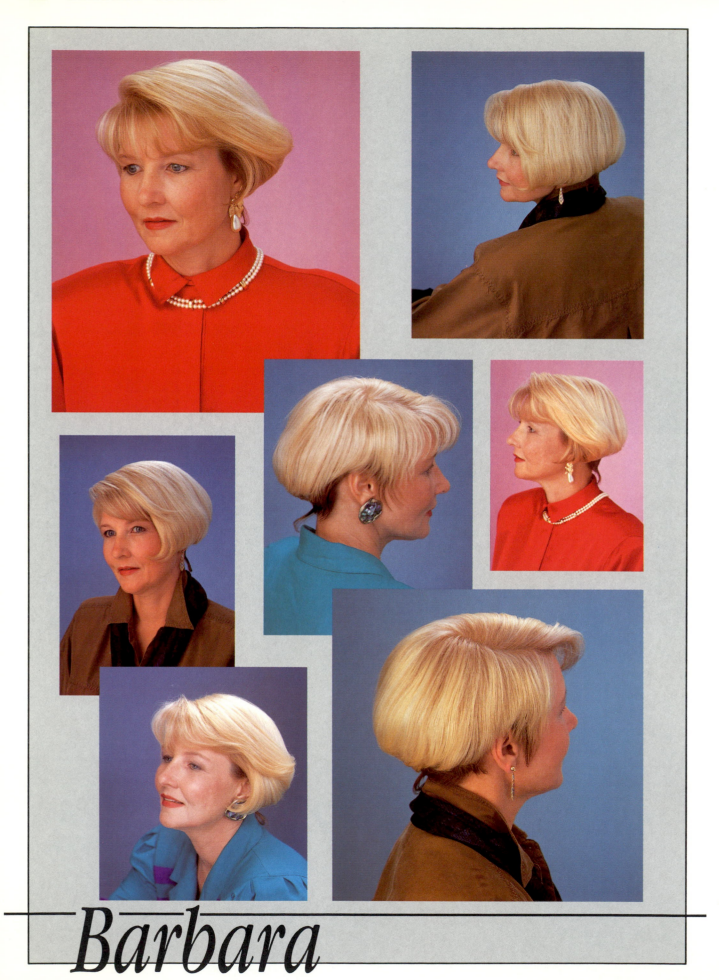

Barbara

Three Colors – Surface Lights

ALTERNATION — LIVELY REDDISH-BROWN

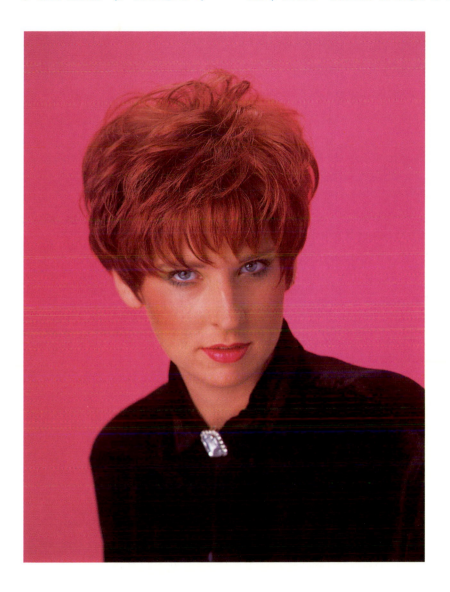

Short hair is more interesting if varied light reflection creates the illusion of undulating movement on an otherwise smooth surface. A visually active surface, created by compatible colors and free-form highlighting, provides softness and an array of colors that complement the client's skin tone and eye color.

A combination of colors used in concert with the client's natural color creates dimension and adds drama to otherwise flat, uninteresting natural tones.

No. 4 *Lynn*

ESSENTIALS

COLOR FACTS   When combining compatible colors, select colors between the lightest possible shade (without bleach) and the client's natural color.

HAIR ANALYSIS   The client's virgin hair color is Level 5 with abundant red tones (dark reddish-brown).

Tonal value: warm

Porosity: good

Texture: smooth

DESIRED COLOR   Subtle color change that gives highlights and artistic interest to a dark, layered form. The client's skin tone is olive; eyes intense blue-gray.

FORMULA 1   2 oz. Level 5 (dark copper)

2 oz. 10-volume (3%) peroxide or developer

FORMULA 2   Powder bleach mixed with 20-volume (6%) peroxide to paste consistency

FORMULA 3   2 oz. Red Currant Surface Stain

PROCEDURE

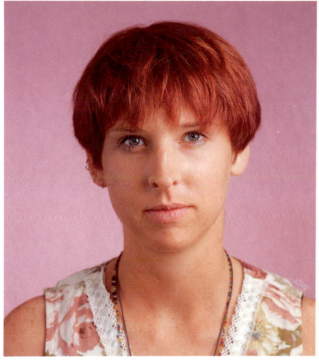

1 The natural hair as it appeared before color-lighting

2 Apply Formula 1 (dark red) to the entire head. Allow it to process 30 minutes or according to manufacturer's directions.

When the processing is complete, remove the tint, rinse the hair and towel-dry to remove excess moisture.

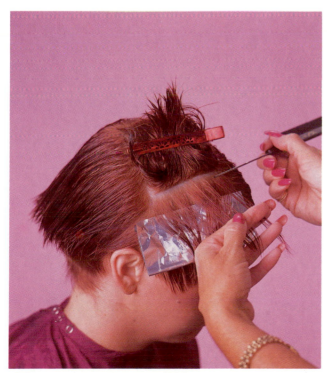

3a Starting with upper crown, slice and weave out a narrow section of hair.

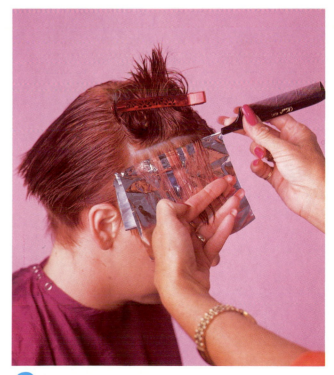

3b Slice and weave.

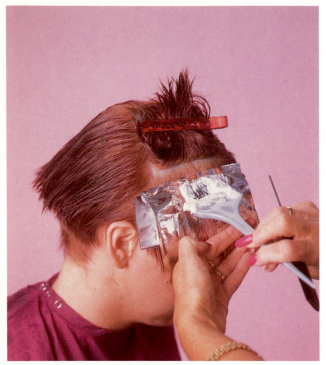

3c Slide a foil strip underneath and brush on a thin layer of bleach mixture (Formula 2).

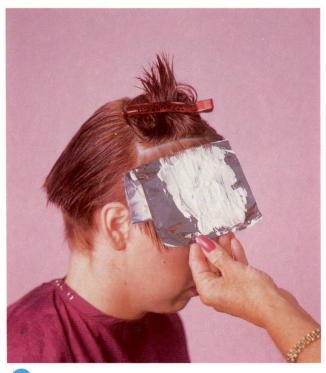

3d After the bleach has been brushed on

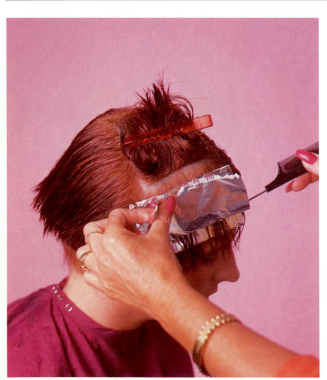

4 Fold the foil from ends toward the scalp, enclosing the bleach. The depth of color removal can be controlled by the volume of peroxide used.

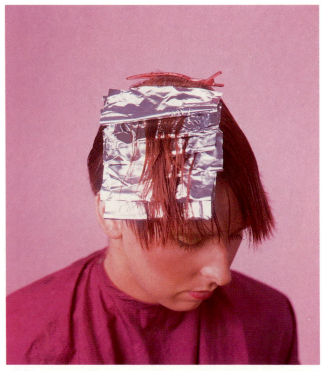

5a Continue to slice, weave out, and foil narrow sections of hair throughout the crown.

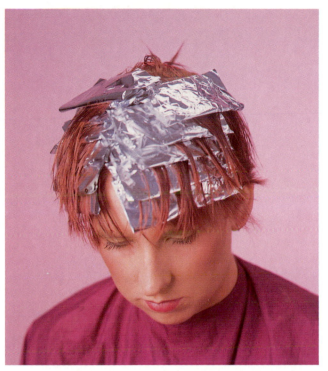

5b Alternate the application so every third slice is the darkest red shade (Formula 1).

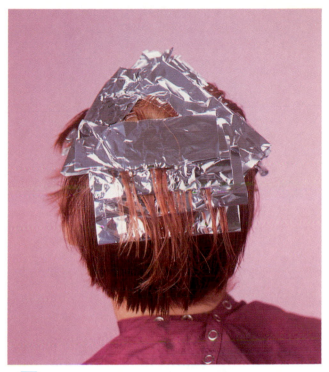

5c Continue over the natural curve of the head.

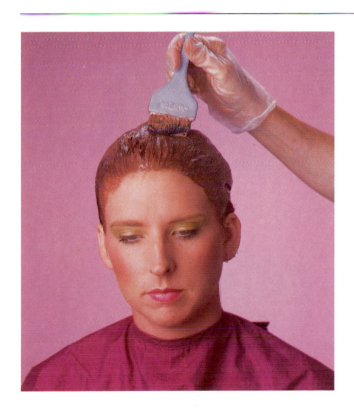

6 When the color has been lifted approximately two shades, remove the bleach, rinse the hair thoroughly, towel dry and apply Formula 3 (Red Currant) to the entire head. Process according to manufacturer's instructions.

The hair is now noticeably alive with vibrant, compatible shades of color ranging from warm reddish-brown on the inside to brick-red surface shades. See finished styles (montage).

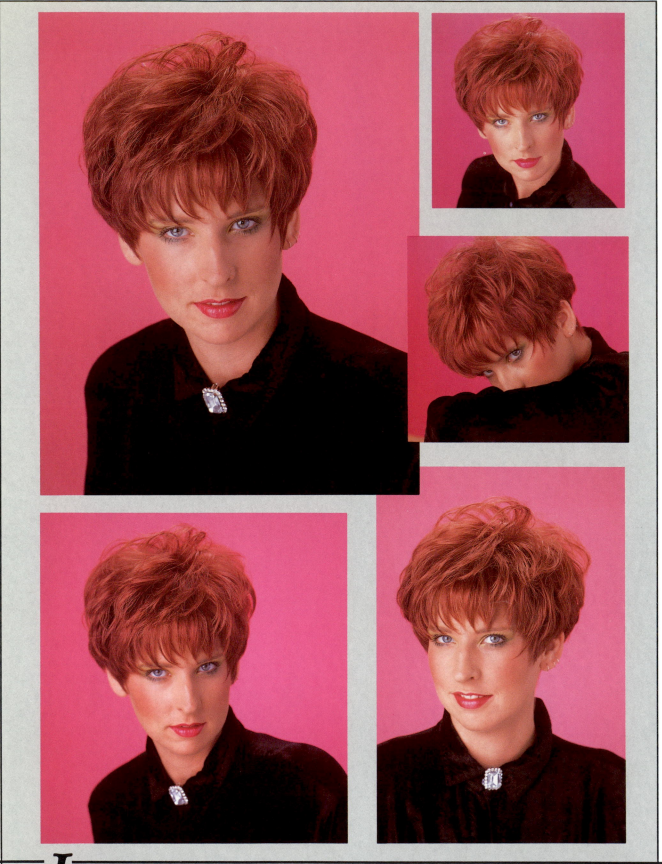

Lynn

Four or More Colors

PROGRESSION OF COLOR

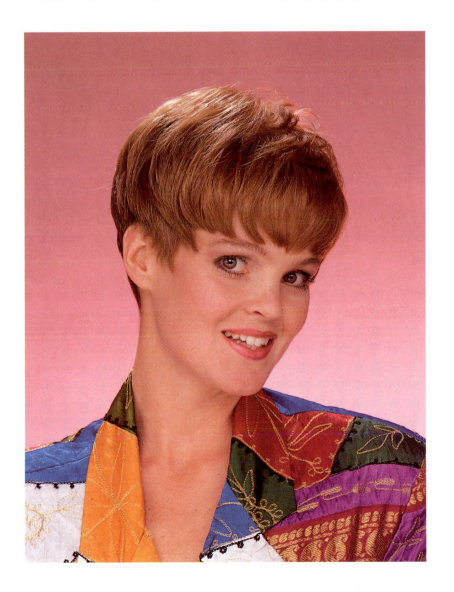

A progression of hair colors — from light to dark or dark to light — along ascending or descending style lines can accent good facial features or diminish those that are less than perfect. Color progression consisting of four or more colors can create directional and dimensional effects.

No. 5 *Linda*

ESSENTIALS

COLOR FACTS

The most contrasting colors should be used at both extremes. Colors used to move from one shade to another must be gradual. No more than a two-shade difference should be used side-by-side.

The best visual effects can be achieved by using colors with equal tonal values — all cool or all warm.

HAIR ANALYSIS

Natural hair color is Level 6 (light brown) with Level 7 highlighting.

Tonal value — warm

Porosity — medium porous

Texture — normal

DESIRED COLOR

Due to the client's skin tone and short hair style, the technician and client decided the hair should have subtle, soft red shades.

FORMULA 1

1 oz. Level 6 medium red base — copper glaze

1 oz. 10-volume (3%) peroxide or developer

FORMULA 2

1 oz. Level 7 red-orange base — muted bronze

1 oz. 10-volume (3%) peroxide or developer

FORMULA 3

1 oz. Level 8 red-orange base — honey red

1 oz. 20-volume (6%) peroxide or developer

FORMULA 4

1 oz. Level 9 red-orange base — ripe strawberry

1 oz. 20-volume (6%) peroxide or developer

PROCEDURE

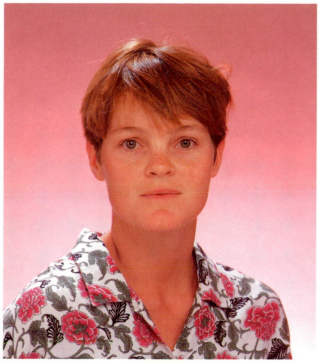

1 The hair color before four-color progression was Level 6 (warm light brown).

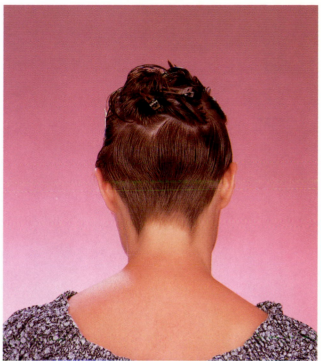

2a To prepare for application, part the hair into four horizontal sections. Zigzag each parting to blend each successive color:
- Ear-to-ear across the occipital bone.

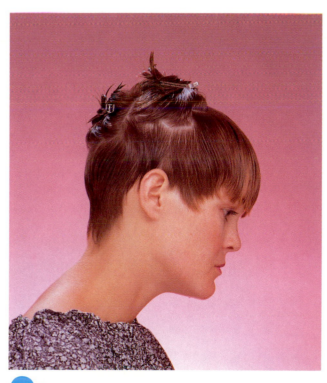

2b
- Ear-to-ear across the lower crown.

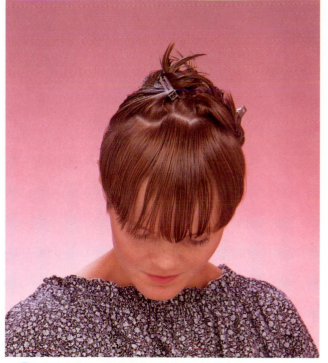

2c
- A part in front of each ear, straight over the head.
- The forward section is the face frame (as wide or narrow as adaptable).

3 Mix the four formulas.

> **Note:** If the technician is skilled at rapid application of hair color, all four formulas may be mixed at one time — in separate containers. The brush must be thoroughly cleansed after each formula or a different brush used for each.

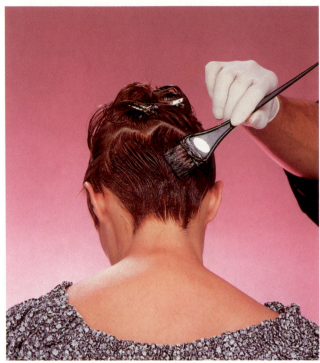

4 Apply Formula 1, the darkest of the four colors, to the nape area. Carefully lay a strip of pliable plastic across the area.

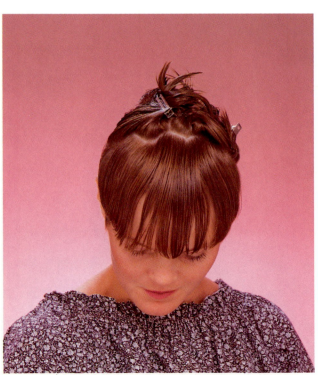

5 Apply Formula 2, Level 7 (red-orange base), to the section directly above the occipital bone. Protect the area with a pliable plastic strip.

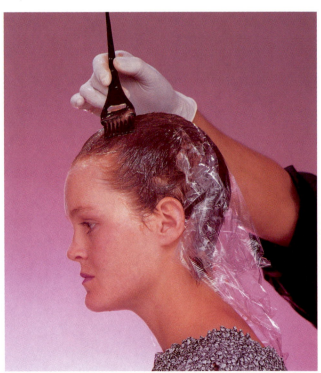

6 Apply Formula 3, Level 8 (red-orange base) to the section over the crest of the head and, like the preceding sections, protect with a strip of pliable plastic.

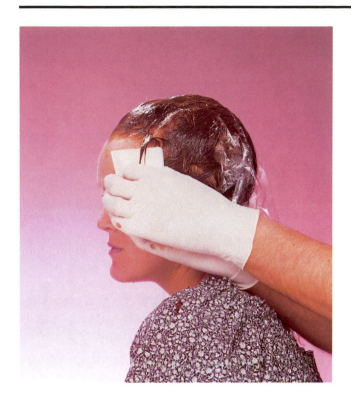

7 The front area (face frame) is the last to be applied. Use Formula 4, the lightest of the four colors — Level 9 (red-orange base).

Allow the color to process for about 30 minutes, taking periodic strand tests on various sections of the hair.

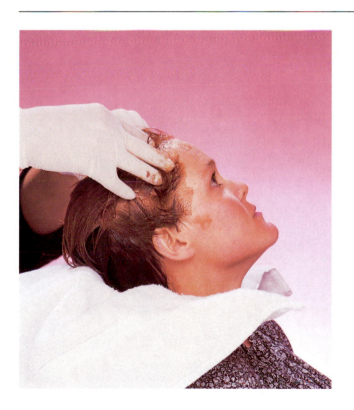

8 At the shampoo bowl, apply diluted shampoo to the hair and quickly blend all colors. Rinse thoroughly with tepid water, directing the spray from front to back. Apply a mild color-formulated shampoo and cleanse the hair once more. Rinse, and condition if necessary.

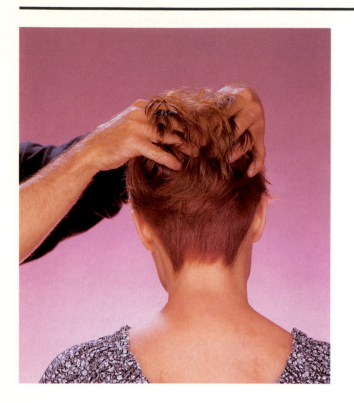

9 Examine the hair throughout in strong, natural light to be sure the colors are subtle and gradually progressive and that warm tones are present.

Note: Since the previously highlighted strands throughout were not filled prior to progressive coloring, additional inner shades could be created due to the variance in the original color.

A variety of undulating colors, each in harmonious concert with the other, create an illusion of vibrance and softness.

This technique lends itself to many styling options. See finished styles (montage).

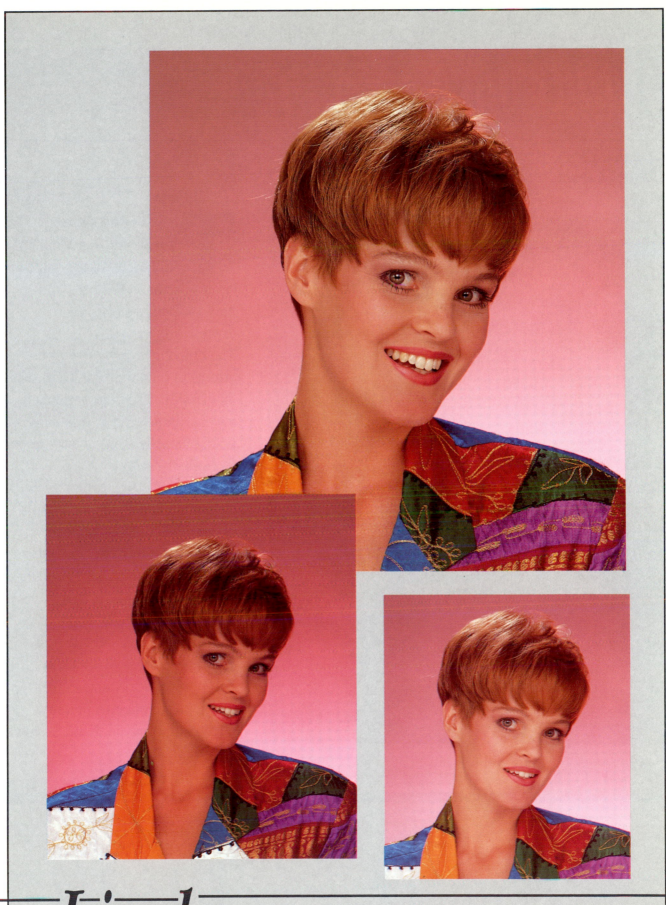

Linda

Dual Colors – Zoning

HARMONIZING LEVELS OF COLOR

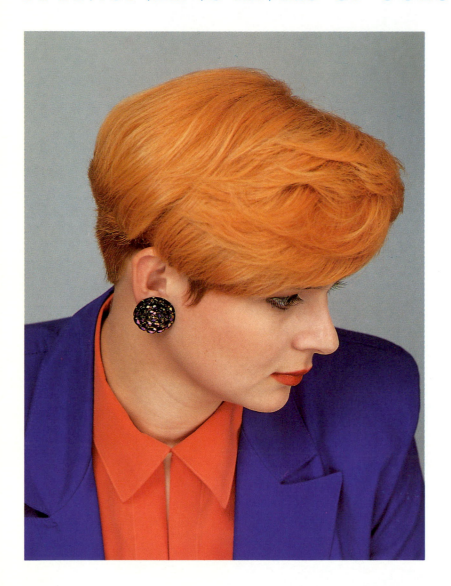

There are no set rules for zoning — adding different color levels to various areas of the hair. You have unlimited freedom of expression.

The object of zoning is to focus attention on particular areas of a hair design. The colors selected may be light or dark, dramatic, bold, or subtle. Taste seems to be the only criterion.

The most effective zoning techniques are achieved when levels of color are used in harmony, as opposed to contrast. There are exceptions to this theory, but when one area of the hair is drastically lighter or darker than surrounding areas, the look is apt to be somewhat shocking. Zoning artistically applied has the opposite effect: a pleasing illusion of movement and design.

No. 6 *Debby*

ESSENTIALS

COLOR FACTS

If the natural hair color has warm tones (red, orange, yellow), as opposed to cool tones (blue green, violet), it is best to select zoning colors that have warm tonal value.

If the darkest desired shade is more than three levels lighter than the natural hair color, consider pre-bleaching all the hair then applying different levels of color over the lightened hair. This would also create an overall iridescent appearance.

HAIR ANALYSIS

The natural hair color is Level 6.

Tonal value — warm

Texture — frayed cuticle due to damage from partial bleach.

DESIRED COLOR

Skin tone and eye color would adapt to warm, light shades of reddish-blonde. The hair has a "forward" design. Client and technician decided to create dimensional levels of apricot blonde.

FORMULA 1

2 oz. creme bleach

2 oz. 30-volume (9%) peroxide

FORMULA 2

2 oz. Level 7 radiant apricot

2 oz. 20-volume (6%) peroxide

FORMULA 3

2 oz. Level 8 reddish gold

2 oz. 20-volume (6%) peroxide

FORMULA 4

1 oz. Level 9 strawberry blonde

1 oz. 10-volume (3%) peroxide

PROCEDURE

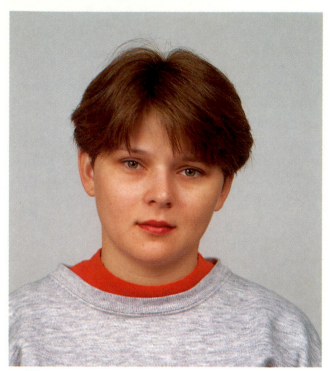

1 The hair before color treatment was a Level 6.

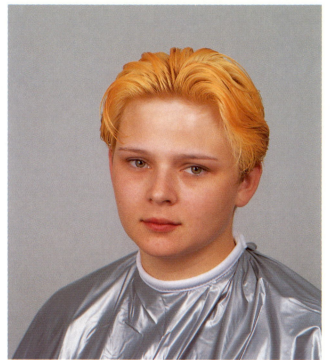

2a Mix Formula 1 (creme bleach). Quickly apply the formula to all the hair (as a soap cap).

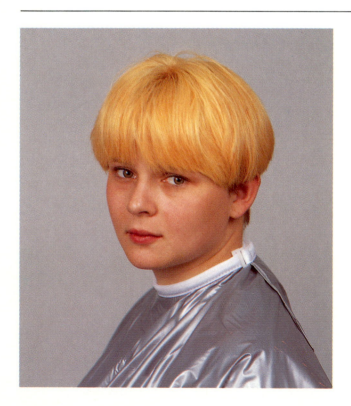

2b Allow it to remain on only until the hair is lifted two to four levels, showing uniformity of color.

Note: When the desired amount of color has been removed, rinse the bleach from the hair and shampoo lightly, being careful not to rub the scalp.

3 Mix the other formulas in separate containers, using a clean applicator brush for each formula.

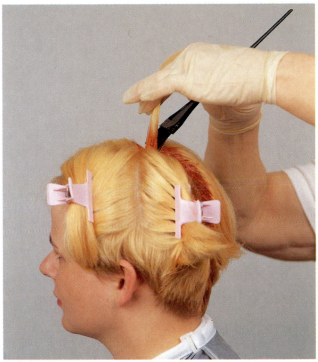

4 Divide the hair into easy-to-handle sections. Starting at the center crown, apply the darkest formula to 1 inch of the hair at the scalp.

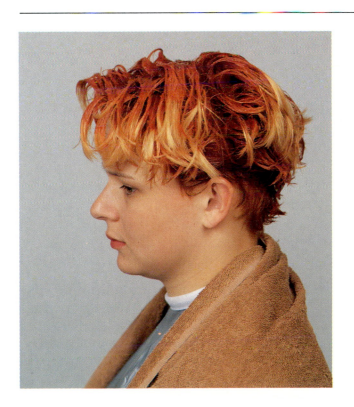

5 Immediately start back over the hair strands and apply the next darkest shade 2 inches down each strand.

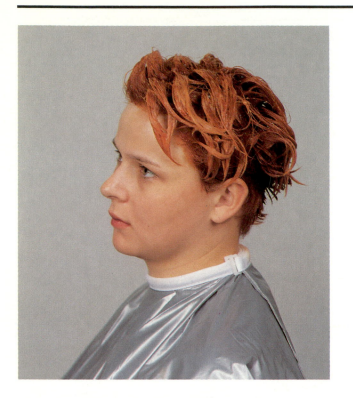

6 Repeat the application procedure, this time applying the lightest formula to the rest of the strand. Allow the color to process 25-35 minutes.

Note: Make no effort to separate the color levels — however, make no effort to blend them at this time.

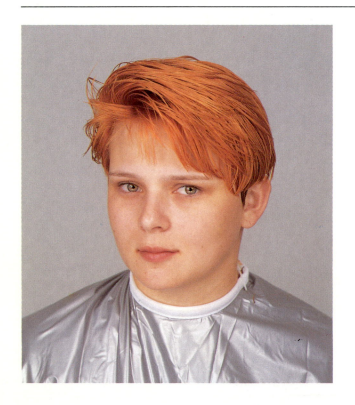

7 Rinse the color formulas from the hair with a strong spray of tepid water. Do not blend the colors.

When the water runs clear, add mild shampoo and lightly cleanse the hair.

The hair should be darker at the root area and gradually lighter toward the ends. This technique looks great when the hair style has a smooth surface. However, it is quite effective for any style.

See finished styles (montage).

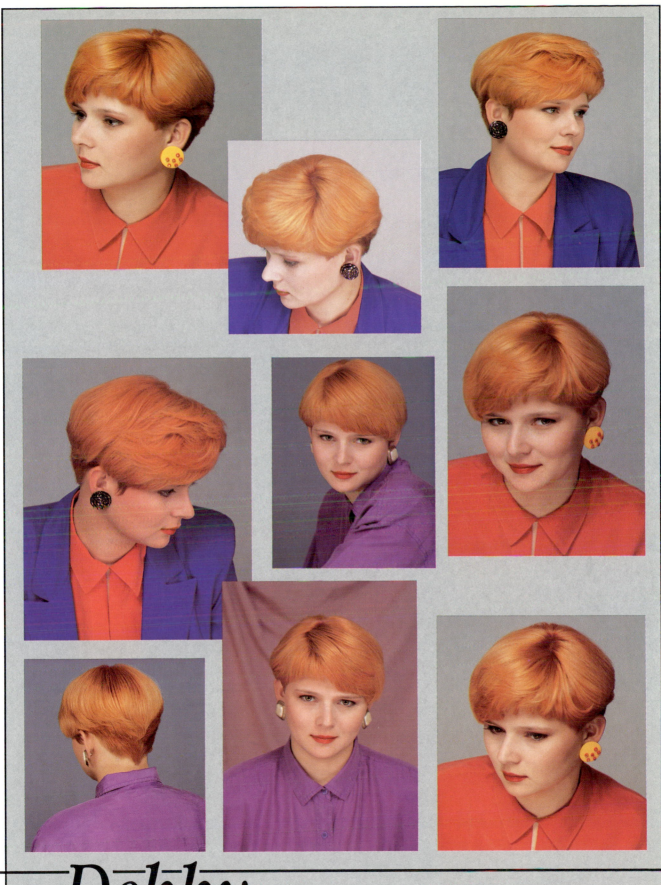

Debby

Three or More Colors – Zoning

CREATING THE ILLUSION OF MOVEMENT

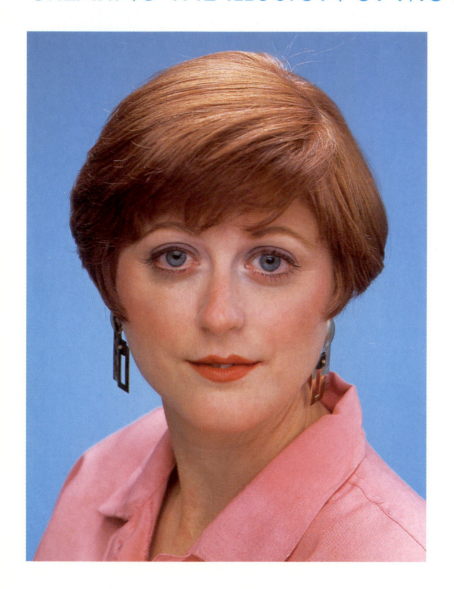

Zoning may be the most creative color application and the most effective way to highlight a focal point within a design.

Zoning procedures may follow the design principles of alternating two or more colors, or the principle of progression may be used. Actually, zoning has characteristics of both inasmuch as multiple compatible colors are used — and they subtly change from one to the other without obvious demarcation. The ultimate guide is individual taste, artistic design, adaptability to facial features, and limitations of the haircut.

A set rule does not govern the application of zoning color. Colors may be brushed on, applied to controlled patterns, or foiled. The end result is limited only by the natural hair color — and the imagination.

No. 7 Pamela

ESSENTIALS

COLOR FACTS

The natural color from which you begin determines color selection, the procedure to be followed, and the results.

For instance, if the original color is darker than Level 5 (medium brown) and you want any zone to be lighter than Level 8 (warm), some of the pigment must be lifted from that zone (bleached).

Hair styles that require the most challenging artistic skills are those that flow forward and closely frame the face. Inevitably, the hair must pivot from some distribution point in the back. That or any pivotal point of a design is an obvious place to position the darkest color from your selections. The following procedure is based on a "forward" design.

HAIR ANALYSIS

Natural hair color — Level 5 (medium brown)

Tonal value — warm

Porosity — medium damage caused by chemical perm

Texture — minimum layers; surface waves

DESIRED COLOR

Eye color and skin tone indicate a color collage in shades of reddish brown, red-gold, and burnished bronze.

FORMULA 1

1 oz. Level 5 reddish brown

1 oz. 20-volume (6%) peroxide or developer

FORMULA 2

1 oz. Level 8 red gold

1 oz. 20-volume (6%) peroxide or developer

FORMULA 3

1 oz. Level 7 burnished bronze

1 oz. 20-volume (6%) peroxide or developer

FORMULA 4

1 oz. Level 8 paprika blonde

1 oz. 20-volume (6%) peroxide or developer

PROCEDURE

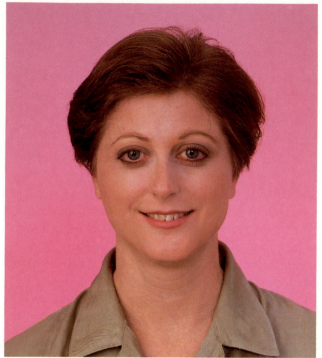

1 Before the zoning color was applied, the hair color was Level 5 (warm tones) without shine.

2 Divide the hair into three definite circular sections. The lower part releases the fringe area at the nape and around the face. The second section is the widest, including all but a 3-inch circle at the lower crown.

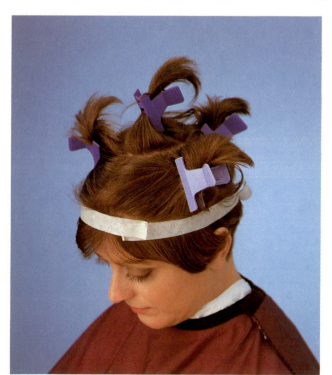

3 Make triangular subsections, each turned in opposite directions, all around the center circular section. Secure each subsection with a plastic holding clip.

4 Mix all four formulas in separate containers. Use a different color applicator brush for each. (Alternate colors are applied very rapidly to the subsections).

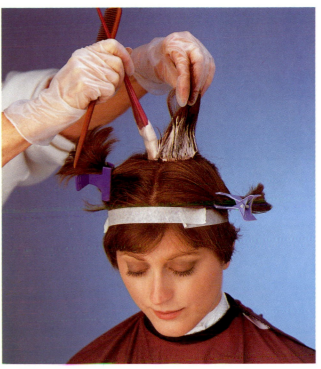

5 Starting with the center circular section, apply the darkest shade to the entire circle.

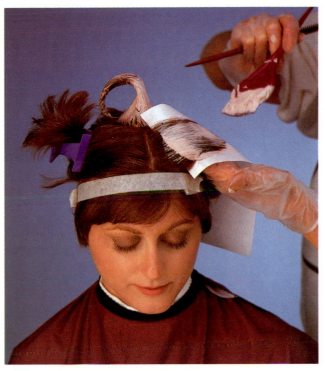

6a Start with the center triangle subsection at the front of the head.

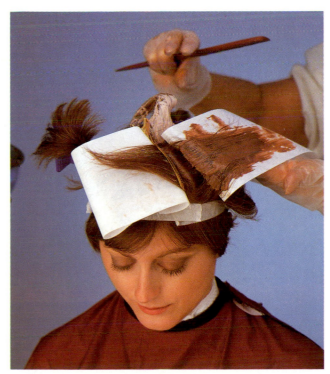

6b Alternate three formulas and apply to subsections.

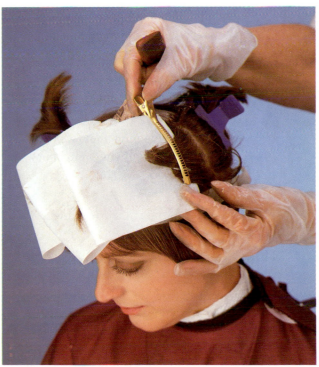

6c Continue completely around the head (separation of colors during processing is not necessary).

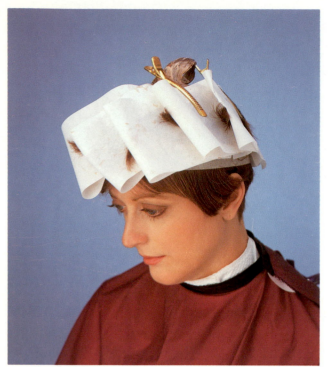

7 Apply the lightest shade to the front fringe area.

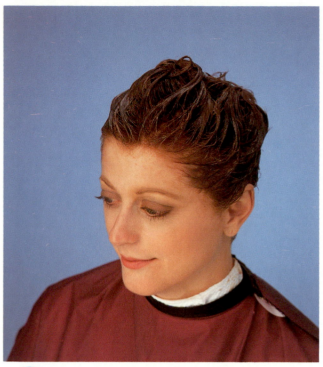

8 Allow the color to process for 25-40 minutes, or until the desired color is achieved.

9 When the processing is complete, mix 1 ounce of the lightest tint used, 1 ounce of very mild shampoo, and 2 ounces of water.

At the shampoo bowl, pour the mixture onto the hair and quickly (a few seconds only) shampoo through the hair, merging all the sections.

Rinse all formula from the hair, shampoo, and use a finish rinse for shine and control.

Move the wet hair in the direction of the desired style. Design the hair to advantageously emphasize the different zones. Styles with a smooth, reflective surface showcase the colors most effectively. Color zoning is one of the most exciting illusions to create with a collage of compatible colors.

See finished styles (montage).

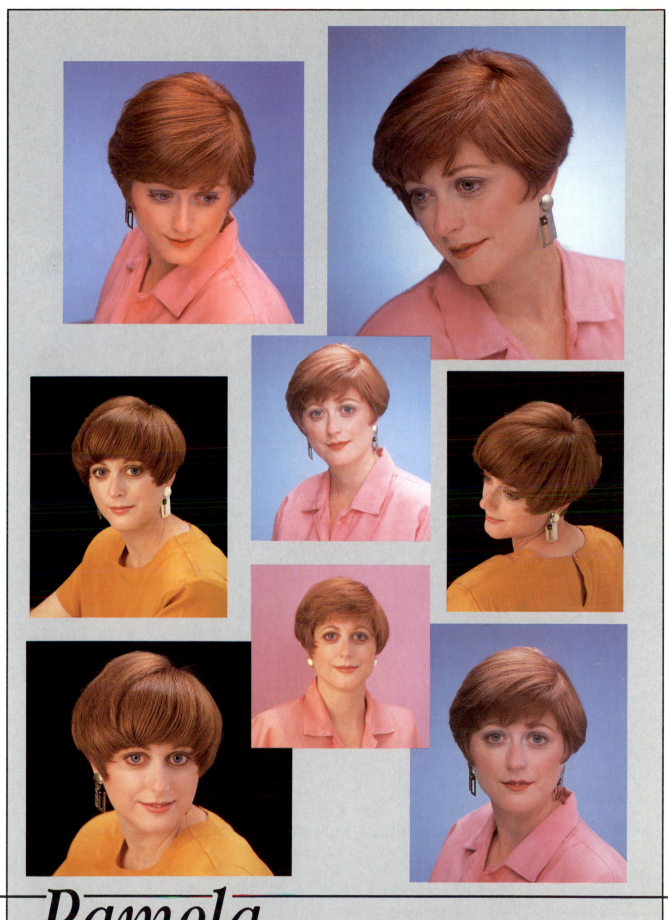

Pamela

Blonde-on-Blonde

DIMENSIONAL HIGHLIGHTING

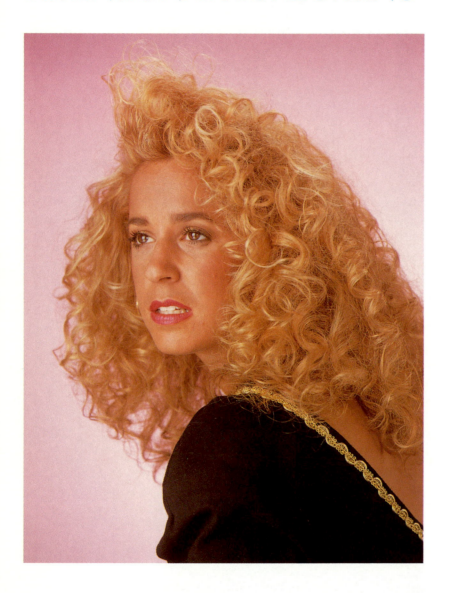

The process of adding or removing pigments from selected strands of hair to enhance or alter natural hair color is known as highlighting. Dimensional color effects can be achieved with several techniques.

No. 8 *Shanna*

ESSENTIALS

TECHNIQUES

The most common technique is *foiling* — selecting, color treating, and isolating the strand by wrapping it in foil.

Foiling requires other techniques when selecting and isolating hair strands to be color treated — namely, *weaving* and *slicing*. The difference in the two techniques is minute, but the end result can vary greatly. The end result of any method of highlighting depends on the size of the strand and the degree to which it is lightened.

Slicing: Release a narrow section (1/16-1/4 inch) by making a straight part at the scalp. Repeat the parting throughout. One or more colors may be used. Natural hair may be left untreated or it, too, may be colored.

Weaving: Using a fine-tail comb, make a definite zigzag part to release a narrow section of hair. Hold the section firmly and slice through the top of the section, isolating only the upper points of the zigzag. The width of the section to be color treated or bleached depends on the desired effect.

POSSIBLE RESULTS

Dimensional effects created by highlighting depend largely on the amount of hair selected for color treatment. Fine strands create an all-over blended appearance. Wider strands will result in a definite color contrast (The color technician is definitely in control of the result).

COLOR FACTS

The color level of the natural hair must first be taken into consideration. In order to create natural looking, well-blended color effects, select color levels not more than four levels lighter than the natural color.

Example: High-lift bleach (complete color removal to Level 10) should only be used on hair with a natural level of 6 or higher. If the natural hair is Level 5 (dark brown), the lightest color used should be no lighter than Level 9 (light golden blonde).

HAIR ANALYSIS

Natural (virgin) hair color — Level 6
Tonal value — warm
Texture and condition — good

DESIRED COLOR

A collage of blonde shades ranging from Level 6 to Level 10.

Note: In order to realize a collage of color incorporating the natural color, at least three levels of color should be used.

FORMULA 1

2 oz. powder bleach
2 oz. 10-volume (3%) peroxide

FORMULA 2

2 oz. Level 9 light golden blonde
2 oz. 20-volume (6%) peroxide

FORMULA 3

2 oz. Level 8 strawberry blonde
2 oz. 30-volume (9%) peroxide)

PROCEDURE

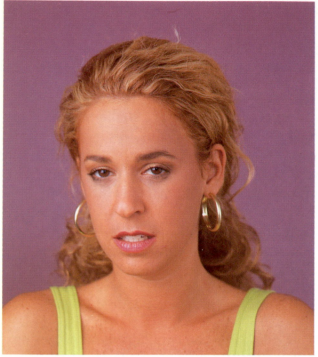

1 The natural hair color, an attractive shade of dark warm blonde, will be considerably enhanced by adding vibrant highlights.

2 Divide the hair into diagonal sections. This allows the hair to be sliced at an angle to the hairline in each section. The color effect is maximized, and no line of demarcation is visible around the hairline.

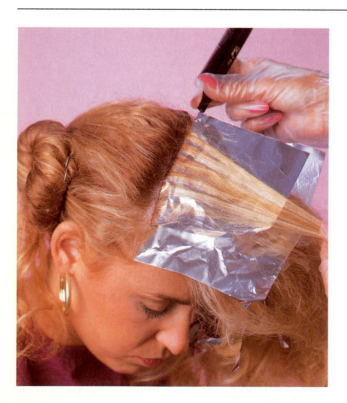

3a Start at the center nape. Slice a narrow horizontal subsection, and place it on a piece of foil slightly longer than each side of the slice, holding it firmly with a tail comb.

Note: Use lightweight foil so it doesn't slip down the hair strand from excess weight.

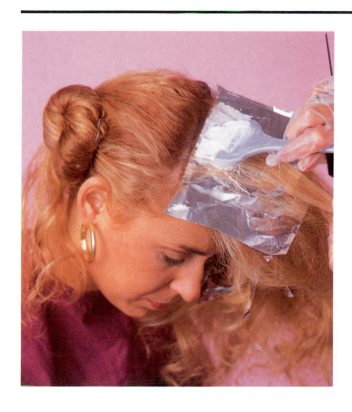

3b Apply the darkest of the three formulas.

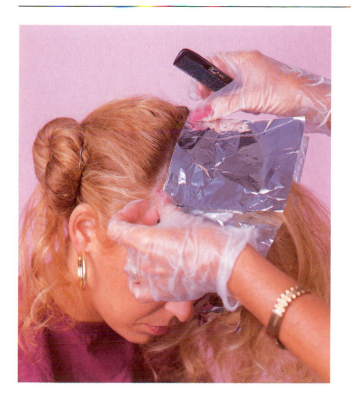

4a Fold the foil on each side and from end to scalp, making a pocket approximately 2 by 2 inches.

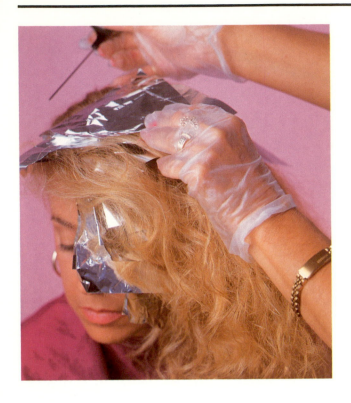

4b Repeat with a slice of the same width immediately above the first, and apply the medium level of the three formulas. Make a third slice the same width as the first two, and apply the lightest formula.

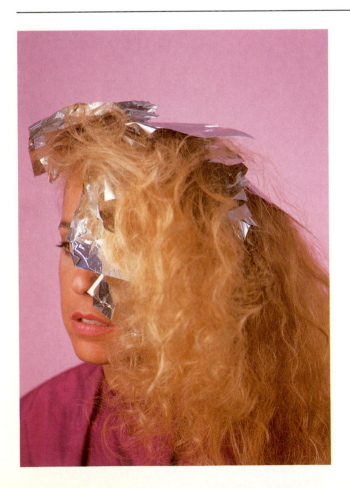

4c The fourth slice (the same width) is left the natural hair color — no color is applied. (Each slice of hair except the natural color is wrapped in foil.) If there is more hair left in the nape section, begin the routine again, applying color in the same order.

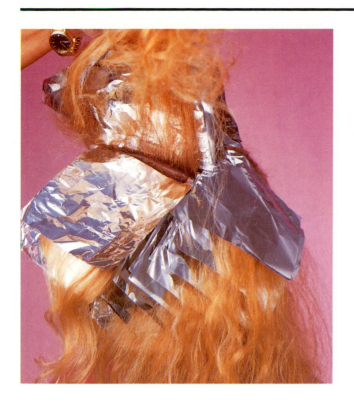

5 Starting at the left side of the center nape and behind the left ear, follow the same procedure used in Steps 1–6, working all the way to the crown.

6 Begin slicing and alternating color formulas on the right side of the center nape and behind the right ear. Work all the way to the crown.

> **Note:** Consider using color-coded foil to keep track of alternate colors.

7 Having finished the back section, start at the left crown where you left off. Alternate the colors with natural hair to the hairline. As you approach the hairline, reduce the width of each slice.

8 Resume working at the right crown. Follow the same slicing procedure, and alternate color application to the hairline.

> **Note:** At this point, only the center front section is left to slice.

9 The center front section may be sliced diagonally to either side or straight from the face. If you opt for straight from the face, start at the back of the section and work toward the center forehead.

10 Allow the color to process. Unfold the foil pockets in different sections of the hair to check the color progress.

When the color has processed sufficiently (usually 25-35 minutes), shampoo thoroughly, rinse, and condition if necessary.

Comb the hair in many directions to examine the color results.

Style the hair suitably for the client

See finished styles (montage).

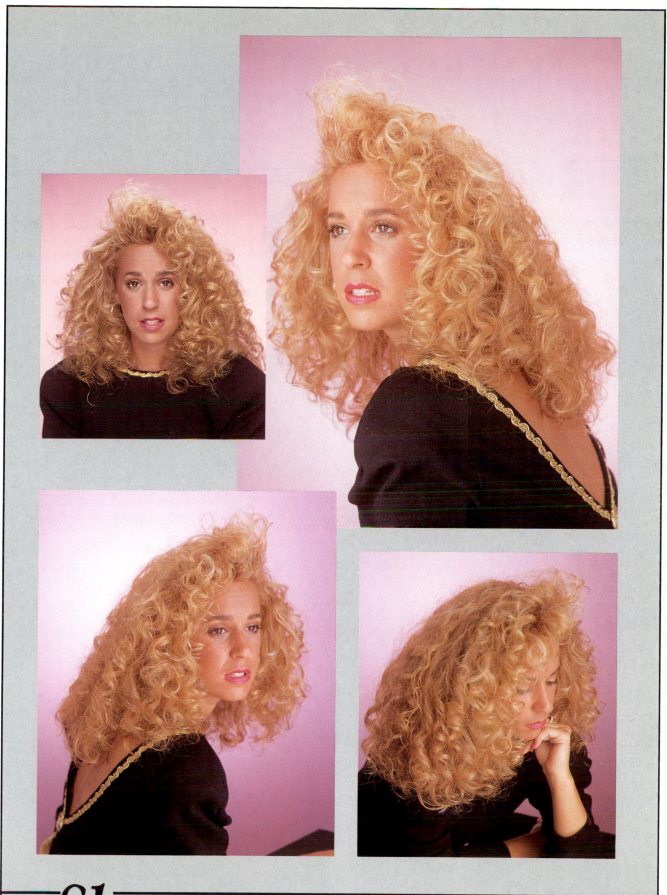

Shanna

Zonal Lighting – Three-Color Tint

FREE-FORM TINTING IN SELECTED ZONES

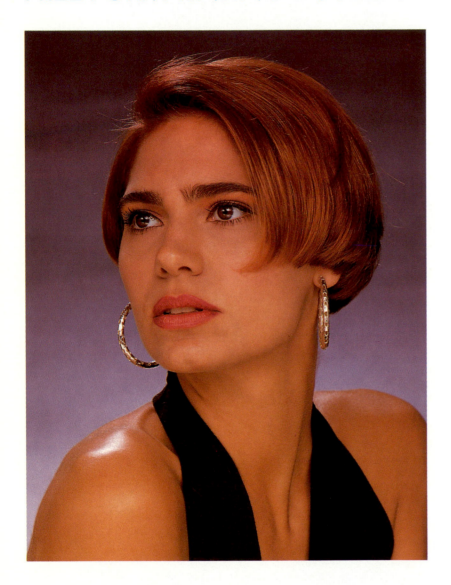

There are no definite rules for free-form tinting other than design principles and the obligatory rule of not mixing cool and warm tones.

Free-form tinting requires a clear design plan with the results in mind. It may help to sketch a pattern so you will know during the application exactly which formula to use in each designated zone.

No. **9** *Kelly*

ESSENTIALS

COLOR FACTS

The ultimate results of a hair-color change, alteration, or touch-up depend on three factors:

1. the color from which you must start
2. selecting the correct formula to attain the ultimate degree of color lift or deposit desired
3. artistic application and correct processing time

Depending on the client's skin tones and face shape, position the lightest (or the darkest shades) so they frame the face. Ordinarily, the lightest shades are used. In this three-color-tint application, the technician determined that the client's features would be most complemented with dark areas at the forehead and nape and the lightest shade cascading over the crown.

For maximum light reflection, the hair style is kept short and straight, with strong directional lines and a smooth surface.

HAIR ANALYSIS

Natural hair color—Level 5 (dark red), faded, and in need of a touch-up.

Tonal value—warm

Porosity—normal

Texture—smooth

DESIRED COLOR

Because the natural hair is all one color, lending no interest or contrast to the skin tone and facial features (see Procedures, Step 1), the desired effect is multiple harmonious levels of red.

FORMULA 1

1-oz. Level 4 red ginger

1-oz. 20-volume peroxide

FORMULA 2

1-oz. Level 7 red gold

1-oz. 30-volume peroxide or developer

FORMULA 3

1-oz. Level 8 bright flame

1-oz. 20-volume preoxide or developer

PROCEDURE

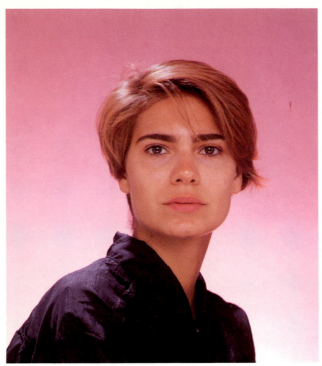

1 The natural hair — all one color, lending no interest or contrast to the skin tone and facial features

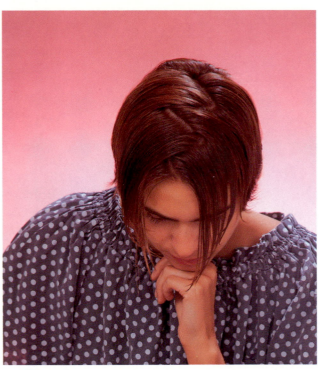

2 Make a zigzag part from crown to forehead as a guide for free-form application.

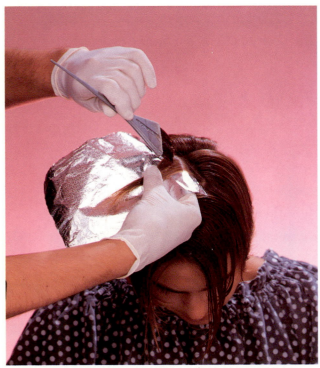

3 Start at the center crown. Section off a 2-inch rectangular portion of hair, and apply the lightest of the three formulas over foil.

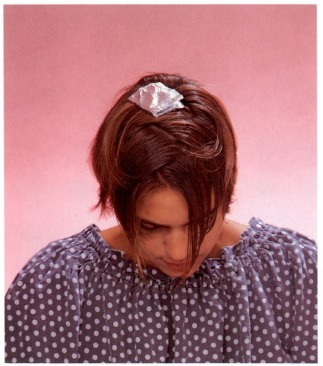

4 Fold the foiled section and use as a guide to continuing application.

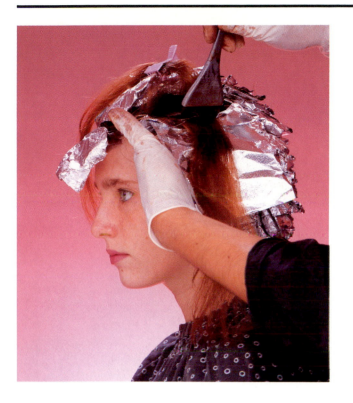

5 Work systematically down each side, in the back over the occipital bone and in the front. Alternate each formula, making sure the darkest formula is nearest the face.

Note: For this client, the darkest formula is applied to the nape area and to the fringe around the face.

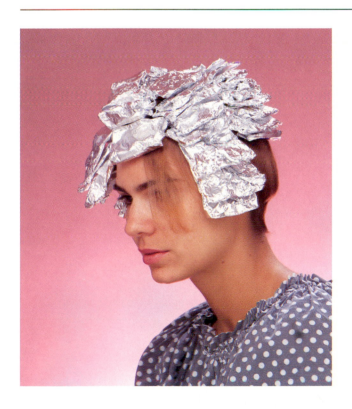

6a Leave natural strands un-foiled at the hair line in preparation for the darkest formula application.

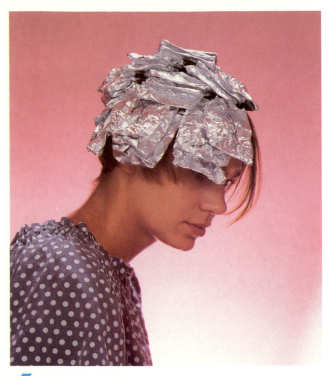

6b Natural strands un-foiled at the hairline

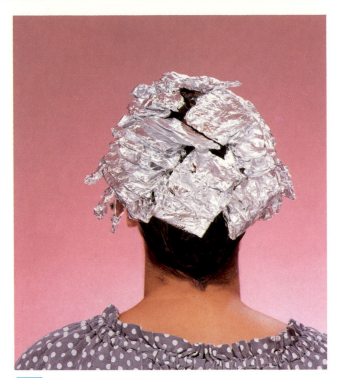

7a Allow the tint to process 25-40 minutes.

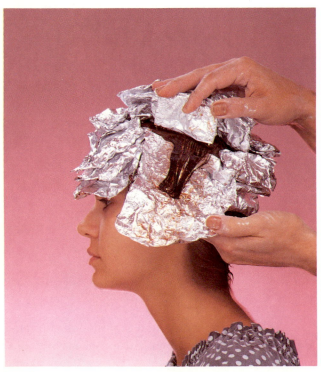

7b Take strand tests at regular intervals to determine progress.

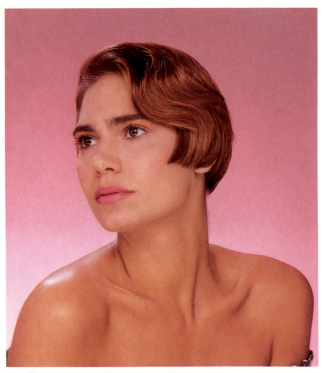

8 The exotic red shades can easily be seen even when the hair is wet.

9 The finished result is more than gratifying (see montage). Excellent reds are often the most difficult to achieve and even more difficult to maintain — but when you please a red-headed client, she is a loyal follower.

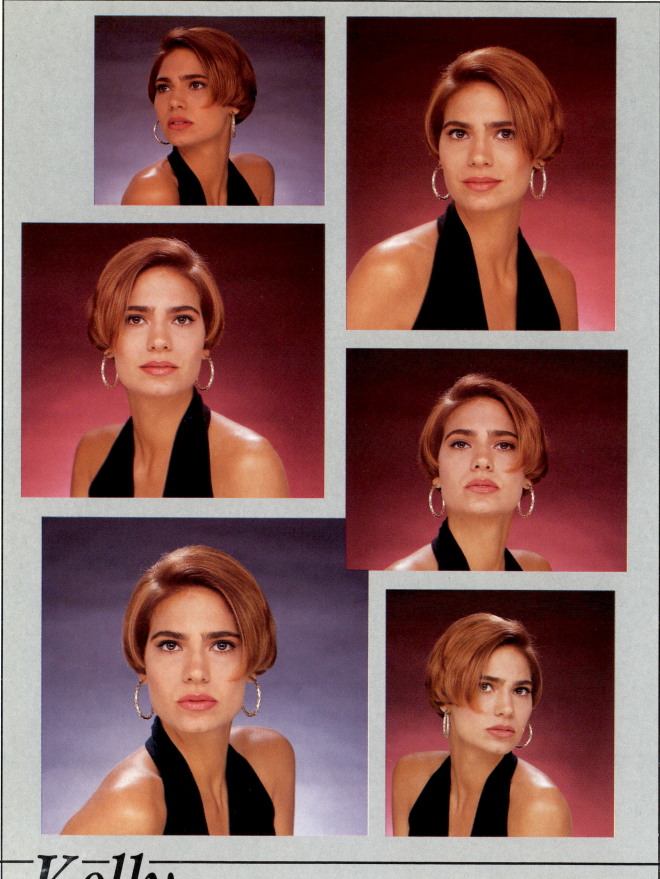

Kelly

Highlighting – Three or More Colors

WEAVE AND FOIL

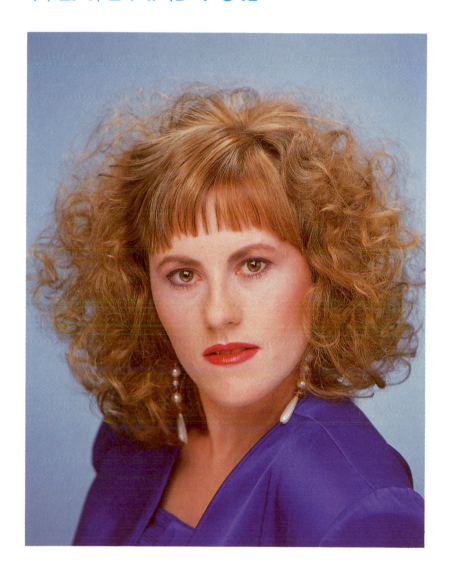

Highlighting and lowlighting are common terms for dimensional hair coloring, also referred to as off-the-scalp color treatment. This is probably the most popular technique in most salons.

Highlighting can be used successfully on a great number of clients, for a variety of reasons. Most often, it makes hair of almost any color level look brighter, but natural. Also, the upkeep is far less demanding than a standard bleach or tint, where new growth is obvious in a relatively short time.

No. 10 *Tommi*

ESSENTIALS

TECHNIQUES

There are two typical techniques of preparing hair for foiling, but weaving is used most often because the colors are more easily integrated and color changes are less obvious as the hair grows out.

Weaving can be achieved with several techniques; for example:

1. Release a half-inch section of hair with a straight part, then weave through the top part of the section to the desired depth. Only the woven strands are color treated and foiled.

2. Release a half-inch (or less) section with a zigzag parting, then select the strands to be color treated by making a straight part through the top of the section, picking up the points as deep or as shallow as you wish.

The amount of hair selected for each foil depends largely on the density of the hair and the desired effect. Ordinarily, finer, more narrow sections create a well-blended appearance. Wider sections tend to create more obvious color changes.

Note: If the hair is long, it may be unnecessary to highlight the area in the back below the occipital bone. However for short hair styles or medium bobs the effect is more pleasing if the hair is also color treated at the nape.

COLOR FACTS

Because a percentage of the natural hair color will be part of the overall finished appearance, it must be considered when selecting three or more colors to create highlights and lowlights. It is suggested that you use two colors lighter than the natural color level and one or two colors darker. When the colors are alternated, the result will be more natural.

HAIR ANALYSIS

Natural hair color — Level 7 (medium golden blonde)

Tonal value — warm

Porosity — good

Texture — medium-fine hair that lends itself best to styles with maximum curl

DESIRED COLOR

Several levels of blond, ranging from pale (Level 10) to dark blonde (Level 6) with warm golden and strawberry accents.

FORMULA 1

1 oz. creme bleach
2 oz. 30-volume (9%) peroxide (Level 10)

FORMULA 2

1 oz. Level 9 pale golden blonde
1 oz. 20-volume (6%) peroxide

FORMULA 3

1 oz. Level 6 medium-dark blonde
1 oz. 10-volume (3%) peroxide

PROCEDURE

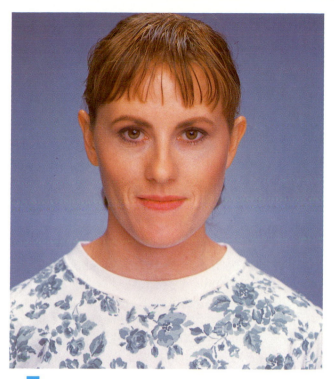

1 The hair before it was highlighted

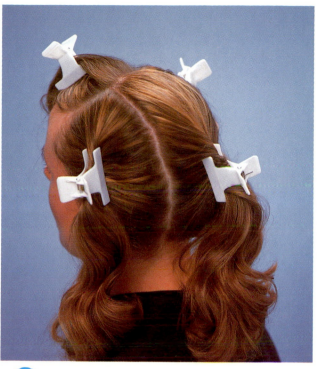

2 Divide the hair into easy-to-handle panels throughout.

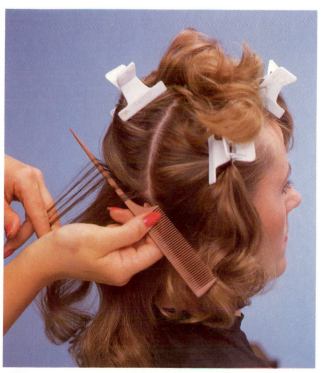

3a Start at the center nape about 2-3 inches above the hairline.

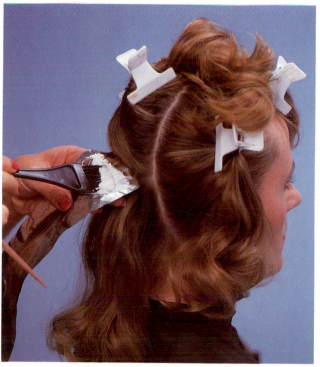

3b Weave a section of hair; place a pre-cut piece of lightweight foil under the section as close to the scalp as possible. Apply the darkest of the four formulas.

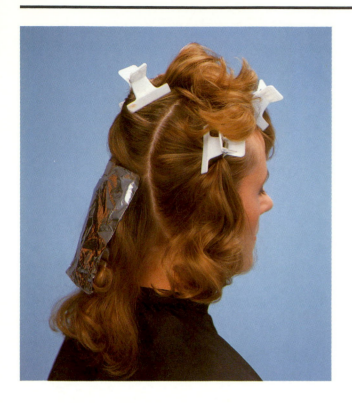

4 Fold the foil from the sides and from the ends to make a pocket.

Note: Fold the foil over the end of a tail comb and hold it firmly under the woven strands.

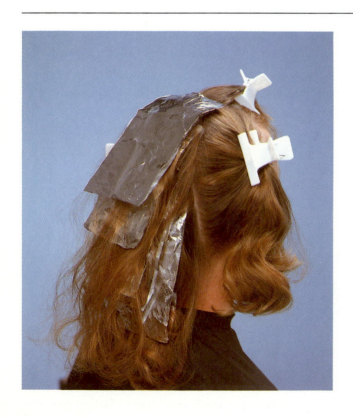

5 Repeat the procedure to the crest of the head, alternating color formulas. Suggested alternation: dark to light, followed by light to dark, then repeated. The color changes will be subtle and will look natural.

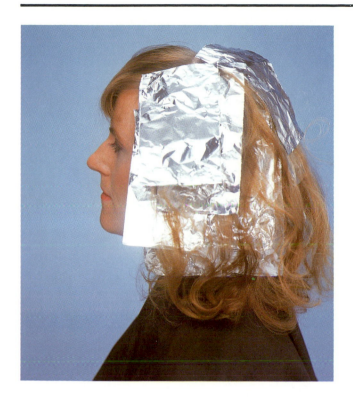

6 When all three panels in the back are finished, weave and foil each side and the temple areas, again alternating hair-color formulas as they were alternated in the back.

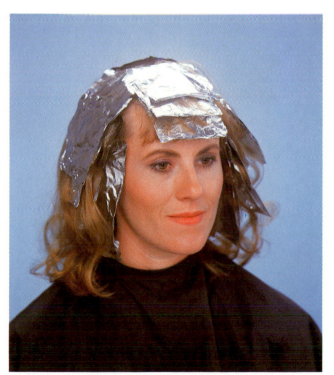

7 Continue from the center crown, center panel, working toward the face frame.

8 Allow the color to process to the levels desired, taking frequent tests, especially on the lightest foils.

When the color has processed to its full potential, shampoo the hair and prepare it for styling.

See finished styles (montage).

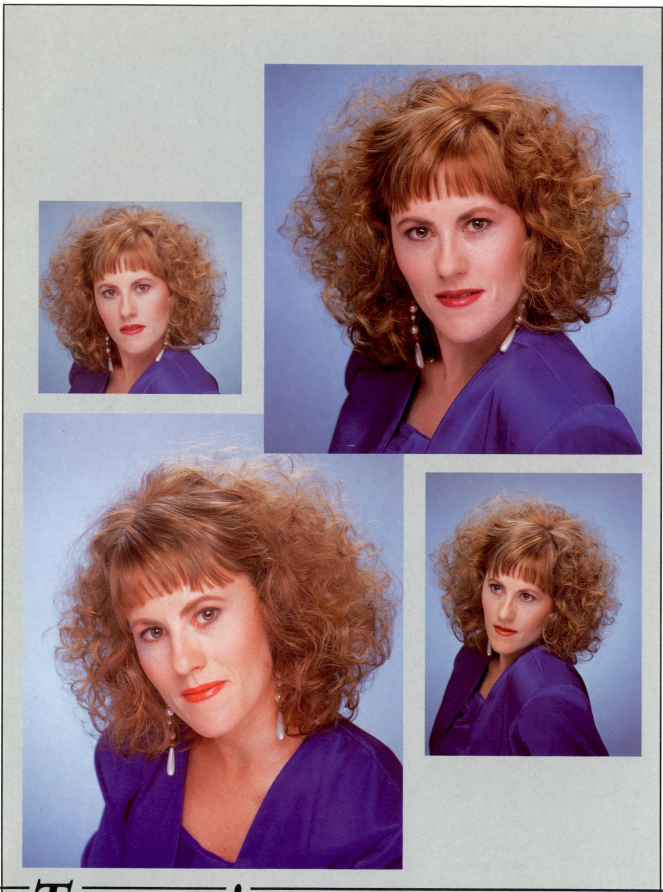

Tommi

Accent Lighting – Sunburst

ISOLATING AND LIFTING COLOR

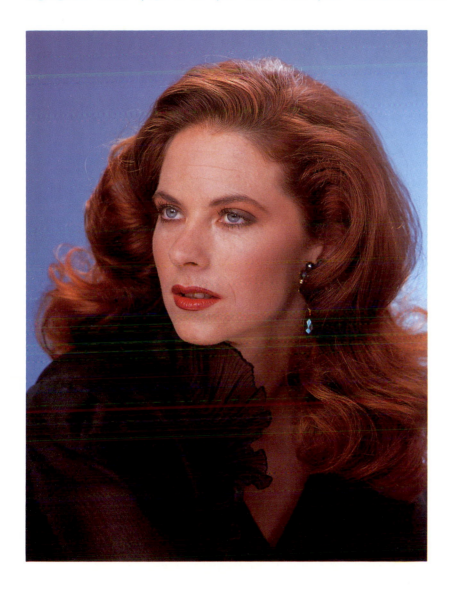

Shades of red are perennially fashionable, but red hair is not for everyone. When selecting a red color for your client, you must take into consideration her skin tones. If the skin tone is cool, shades that fall into the orange end of the color spectrum are not as flattering as colors that fall into the red-purple end.

For that reason, it is easier to accent rich, red colors with various compatible colors. Red-orange lights can be added even if the skin is cool, provided they do not dominate the overall look. If the skin tone is warm, almost any shade of warm red looks great.

No. 11 *Kyle*

ESSENTIALS

TECHNIQUE Several techniques may be used to add accent lights to any hair color. However, a special technique of isolating and lifting color from selected strands during the tint process is very effective.

COLOR FACTS The desired color(s) must be based on the natural hair color. If a portion of the natural hair is to be left natural, becoming a part of the finished color montage, then all colors must be selected to complement the natural color.

When mixing red shades, it is recommended that you darken or lighten the hair within a range of not more than three levels of color.

HAIR ANALYSIS Original hair color — Level 5 (reddish brown), colored on a regular basis to a shade of red

Tonal value — warm

Texture — slight damage requiring a protein conditioner one week before color application

DESIRED COLOR A collage of red shades from levels 5-8. The desired base color is Level 5 (coppery red), with the lightest shade Level 8 (vibrant orange-red).

FORMULA 1 2-oz. intense copper

2 oz. 20-volume (6%) peroxide

FORMULA 2 2 oz. red-gold

2 oz. 20-volume (6%) peroxide

FORMULA 3 1-oz. reddish blonde

1 oz. 30-volume (9%) peroxide

PROCEDURE

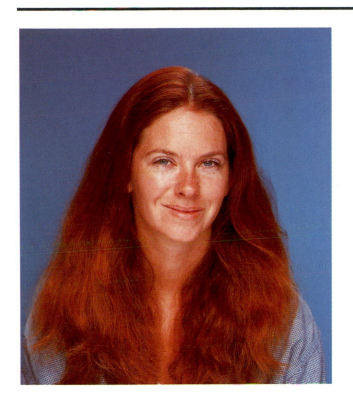

1 Before tinting, the hair was many shades of red with ends several shades lighter as a result of overlapping during retouching.

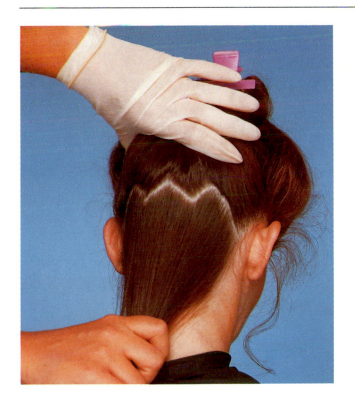

2a Divide the hair horizontally across the head into three easy-to-handle sections. Use uneven parts to avoid lines of demarcation.

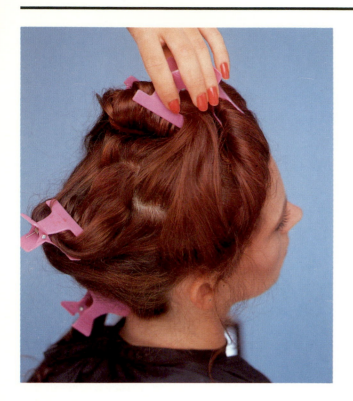

2b Center crown section divided with an uneven part

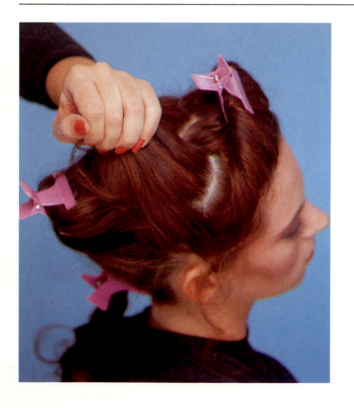

2c Front section divided with an uneven part

Note: When working with very long hair, the lower back section may be applied last so as not to interfere with the sections above until the tint has been applied and the section secured.

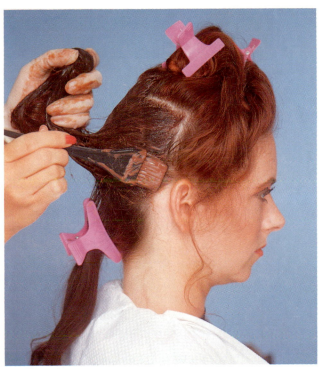

3 Apply the second darkest color (Formula 2) to the center crown section.

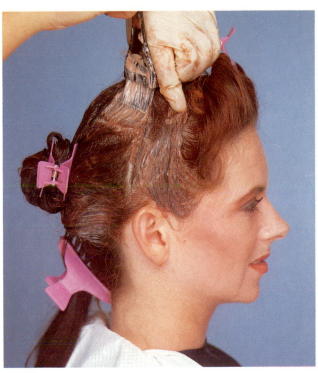

4 Beginning at the temple area, apply the lightest of the three colors (Formula 3) up to the curve of the head on each side.

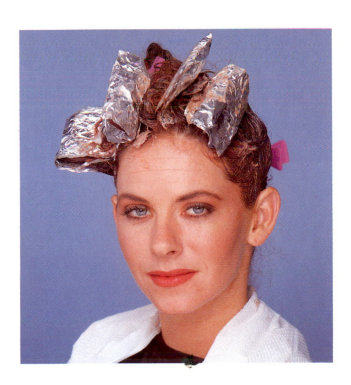

5 In the front section (from one receding hairline to the other), make sections equal in width. Alternate the lightest formula (Formula 3) and the second darkest shade (Formula 2) across that area. Isolate the lightest shade with foil.

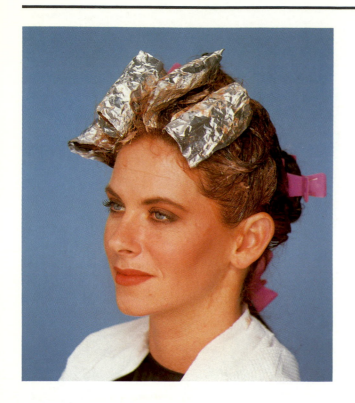

6 Go back through each section to check the coverage, and apply the darkest color to the ponytail at the nape area.

Note: Secure the sections with plastic clips and allow the color to process for 30-40 minutes or according to manufacturer's instructions.

See finished styles (montage).

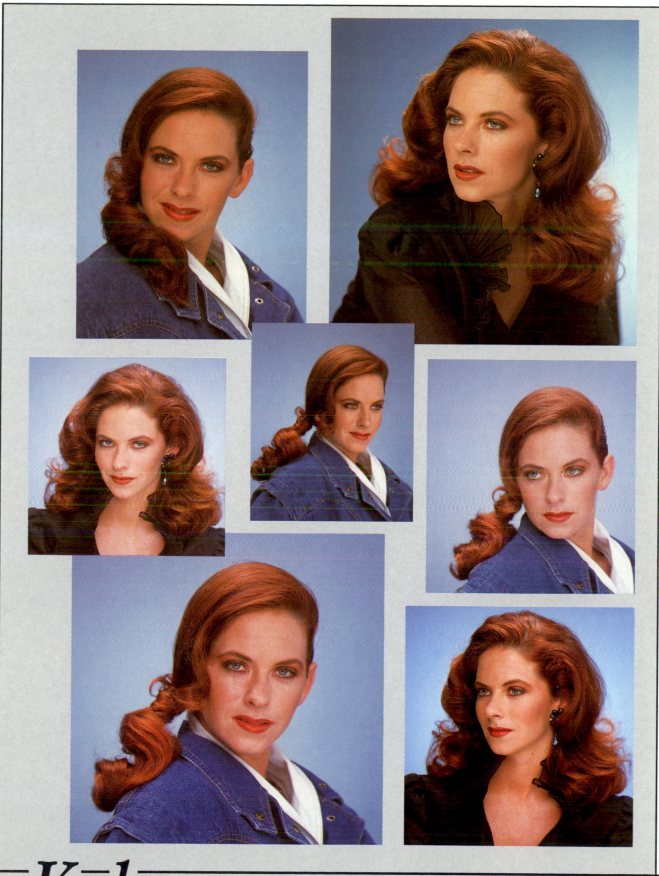

Kyle

Glazing – Surface Color and Shine

NON-OXIDATIVE COLOR

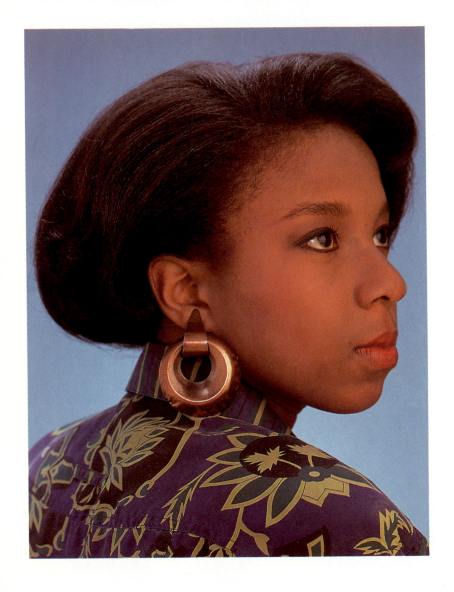

At first glance, this client's hair looks black. But black hair, especially that of African Americans or other people of color, is made up of many shades of brown, red, and gold, predominated by black (levels 1 and 2). In evaluating the colors in predominately black hair, think of specks of color in the iris of the eye. It is important to evaluate those satellite shades in order to select the proper hair-color product and formula that will enhance the surface color and shine.

No. **12** *Carol*

ESSENTIALS

COLOR FACTS
Black hair is best kept in levels 1-3, with intensive surface color added for cosmetic illusion and shine. Because black hair is difficult to lift beyond levels of red, a non-oxidative hair-color product is often chosen over chemically activated products.

Non-oxidative color is an ideal product for hair that has been chemically relaxed or straightened. There is no lifting action; it will not remove color from natural pigment; it will only deposit color, adding depth and tone to existing hair color; it will blend gray or faded hair; and it is gentle on the hair, often containing conditioning properties.

Non-oxidative color stains and seals the cuticle layer of the hair, making the surface smooth and therefore increasing reflecting quality. It gives the appearance of color glaze and ultra sheen.

HAIR ANALYSIS
Original color — Level 2; hair has been chemically relaxed but is in excellent condition.

Tonal value — warm

Porosity — normal-to-slight chemical damage

Texture — excess curl

DESIRED COLOR
The skin tones of women of color vary greatly. The underlying tonal value is either cool (blue/ashen) or warm (gold/red). If gold or red is found mixed into black hair, the skin tone more likely is warm.

To complement this client's warm skin tones, the hair will reflect lights of rich, sunlit brown.

FORMULA
Equal parts of sunlit brown, cinnamon, and ginger

PROCEDURE

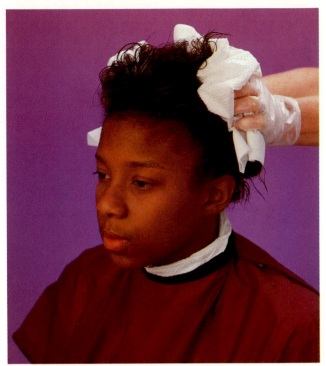

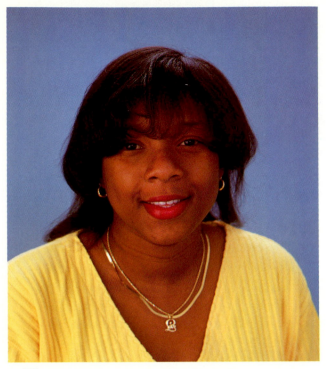

1 The hair color before glazing application was Level 2 (warm).

2 Shampoo and condition the hair. Towel dry until excess water is removed.

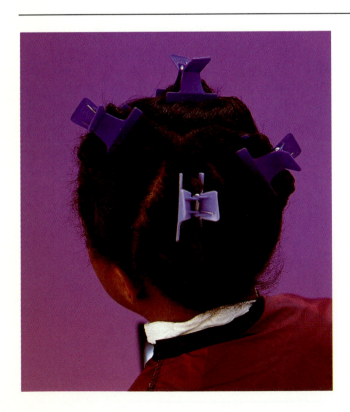

3 Divide the hair into four easy-to-handle sections. Part the hair from center forehead to center nape and from ear to ear over the crest of the head. Secure each section with plastic hair clips.

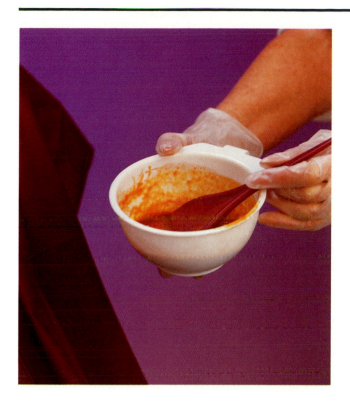

4 Mix the formula in a dish in preparation for application. An applicator bottle may also be used. Since the product is non-oxidizing, it can be applied generously to all parts of the hair at once. The consistency of the product may also be a factor.

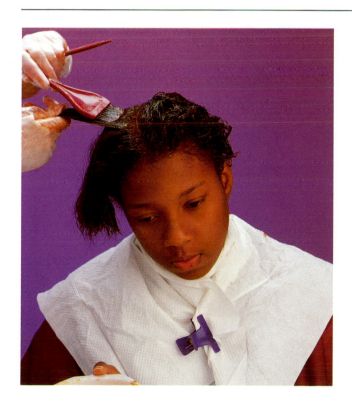

5 Starting at the most resistant area, apply formula to a section at a time until the application is complete.

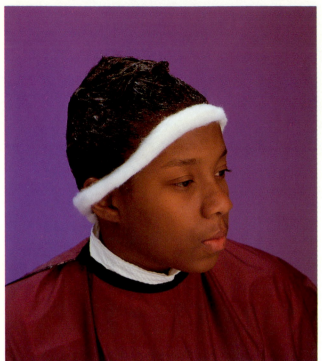

6 Position a strip of cotton around the entire hairline, front, sides, and back. Keep the cotton on the skin, not on the hair.

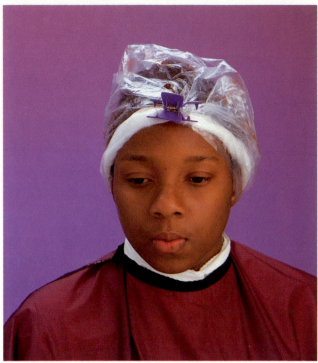

7 Cover the hair and the cotton with a plastic cap or bag, making it airtight. Allow it to process under heat for 30 minutes (follow manufacturer's instructions for timing).

8 When the color has processed sufficiently, rinse thoroughly, gently towel dry, and style as desired.

See finished styles (montage).

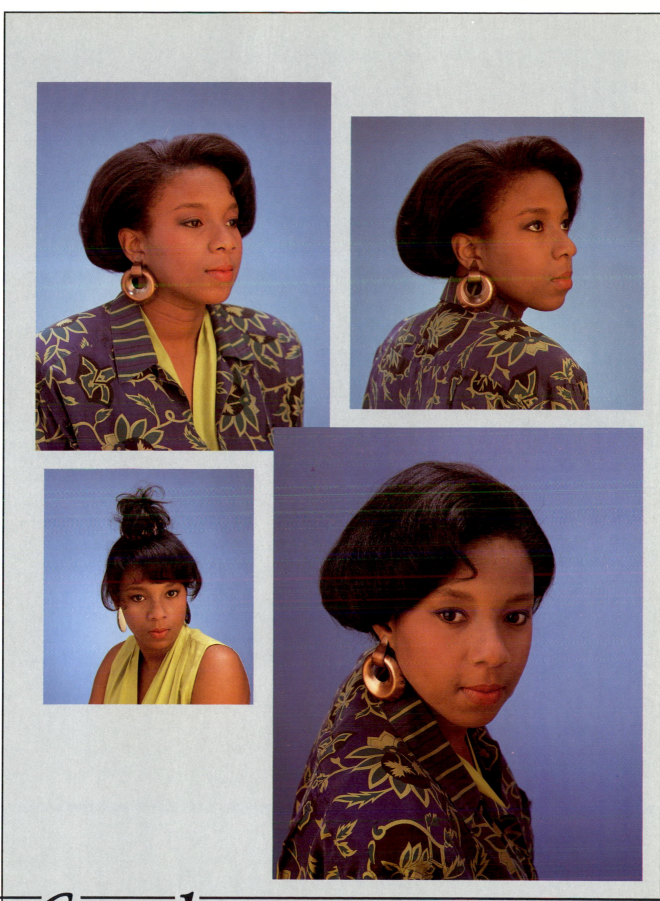

Carol

Icing

COLOR ENHANCEMENT OF BLACK HAIR

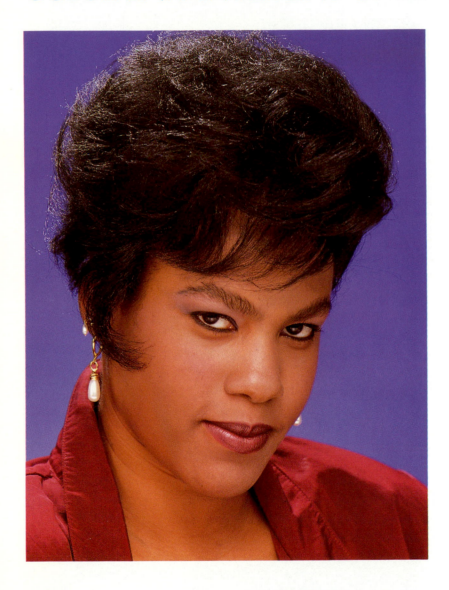

Color enhancement or even a color change can be an exciting option for clients of color who have darkest brown to blackest-black natural hair.

Many African Americans have their hair chemically relaxed. The chemicals in relaxer products increase porosity to a degree that affects the natural strength and elasticity of the hair. This increases the risk of damage from additional chemical hair coloring.

Contemporary hair-color products are safe and effective for any type hair, if the hair is in good condition to begin with and if the manufacturer's instructions are closely followed.

No. 13 Stephanie

ESSENTIALS

COLOR FACTS The darkest hair, Level 1, can be lifted into levels of dark to medium-brown without pre-bleaching. Because black, chemically treated hair is often fragile, pre-bleaching is not recommended.

Porosity is a major factor in controlling color results. Protein re-conditioners should be used to balance porosity for even results.

HAIR ANALYSIS Original hair color — Level 2; ends are (faded) Level 4

Tonal value — cool

Porosity — normal

Texture — natural curl/chemically relaxed

DESIRED COLOR Level 2 (vibrant brown). The skin is medium cool-brown and is best complemented by cool shades of violet, which can be easily attained with cosmetic (non-oxidizing) color products.

FORMULA Equal parts of red violet, indigo, and Blue Mood.

PROCEDURE

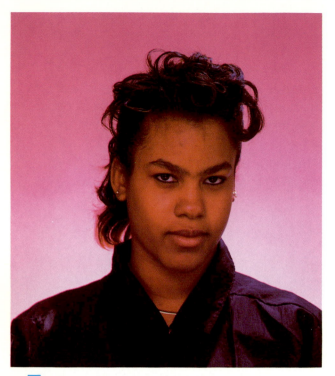

1 The hair before color application.

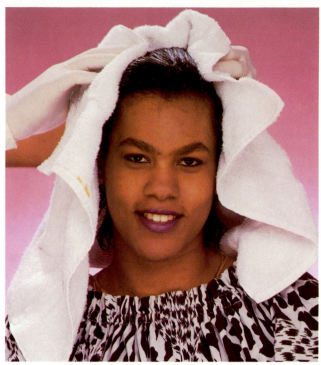

2 The hair must be washed with a clarifying shampoo, rinsed, and towel-dried before color application.

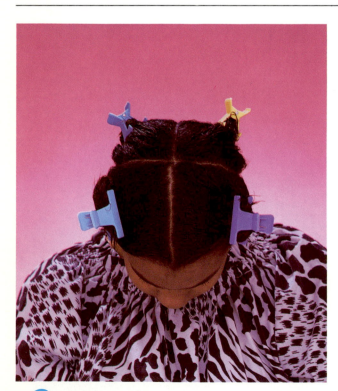

3 Divide the hair into easy-to-handle sections.

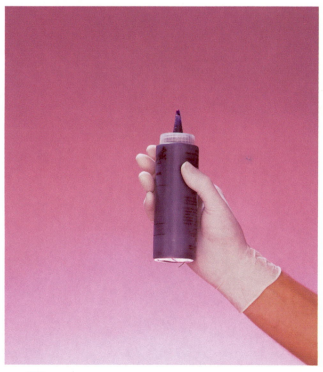

4 Mix all colors together in an applicator bottle for fast, easy application.

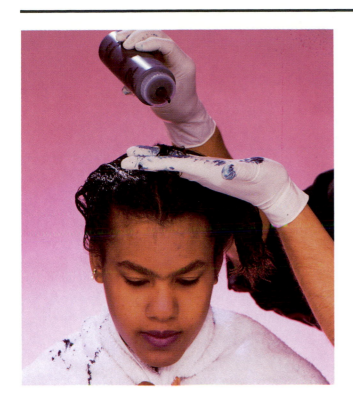

5 Starting at the top of the right back section, make narrow subsections and apply a generous amount of color over the entire head.

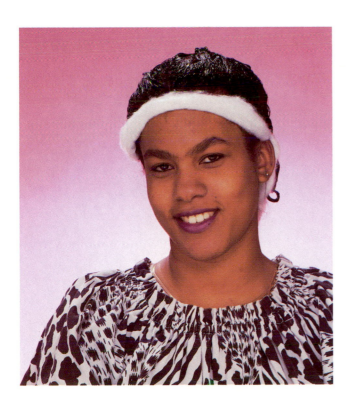

6a Using your finger, rub a small amount of protective cream onto the skin around the hairline, carefully keeping the cream from touching the hair. Place a narrow strip of cotton directly on the skin with protective cream.

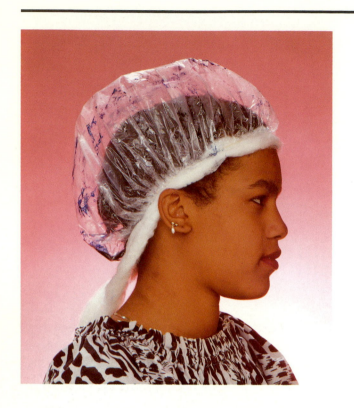

6b   Cover with a plastic cap and process according to manufacturer's instructions.

The results are amazing. The surface of the hair now has a warm, shiny glow.

See finished styles (montage).

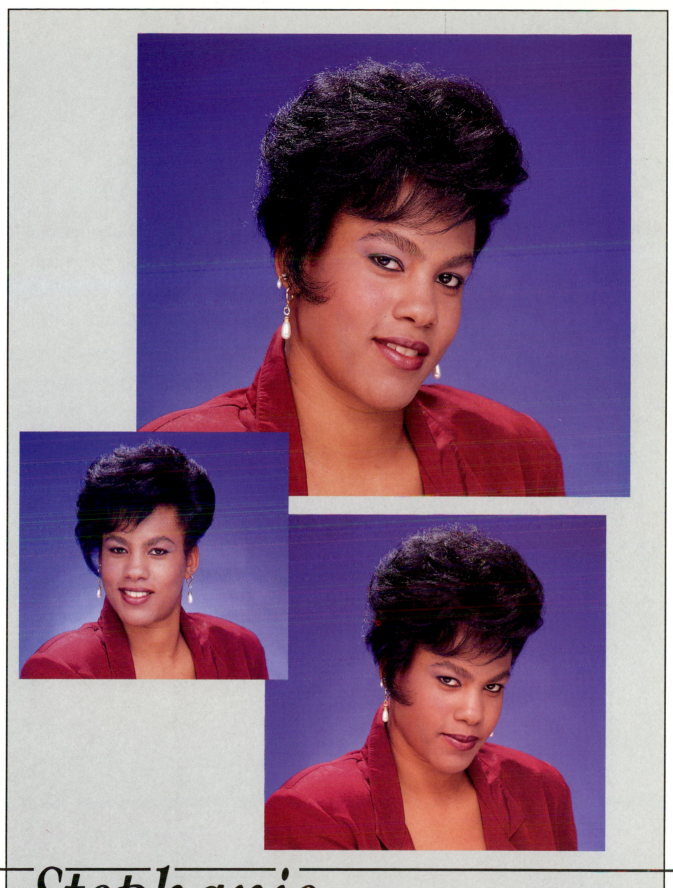

Stephanie

Monochromatic Reds

ADDING DEPTH, DRAMA, AND DIMENSION

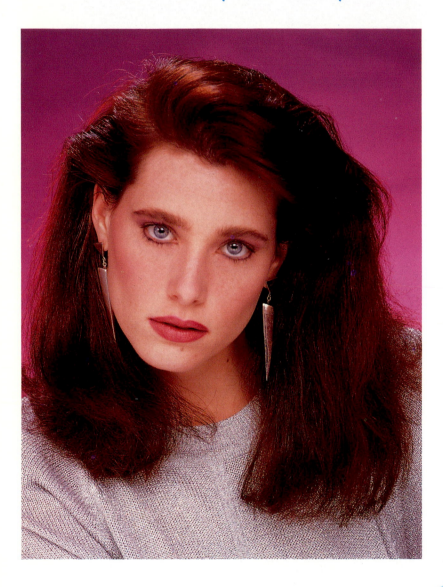

Multiple shades of deep, rich red add dimension and unusual drama to hair of any natural level, but they are most effective on hair levels 5-7. The hair may be color treated overall or on selected areas. The result must be one of harmony by monochromatic illusion.

No. 14 *Sandy*

ESSENTIALS

COLOR FACTS

The predominating rule for determining if red hair will suit a client is adaptability. First, consider the skin tone and eye color. Skin with olive undertones may be more complemented by red hair. Pure brown or deep-blue eyes will both look great with red hair. This color is not recommended for florid skin tones or pale gray eyes. Whether or not the desired color can be achieved depends on color selection as related to the hair color before application.

When selecting red colors, remember that natural hair-color levels 4-7 are likely to contain natural warm tonal value, making red pigments easier to penetrate.

For best results, use hair colors capable of lifting (lightening) the natural hair two to four levels without pre-bleaching.

Although color deposit is more easily regulated, it is suggested that you select colors with enough depth and intensity to complement the lighter colors, producing a subtle monochromatic blend.

HAIR ANALYSIS

Original hair color — Level 5; previously color treated

Tonal value — warm

Porosity — normal

Texture — pre-permed

DESIRED COLOR

Complementary shades of deep, rich red (cinnamon/ginger)

FORMULAS

1 oz. rich cinnamon red — Level 7

1 oz. red currant — Level 6

1 oz. reddish bronze — Level 5

1 oz. reddish blonde — Level 8

Note: Mix each color formula with 1 oz. 20-volume peroxide (6%) or developer of equal strength.

Mix color in separate containers and apply with clean applicator brush or from a clean applicator bottle.

PROCEDURE

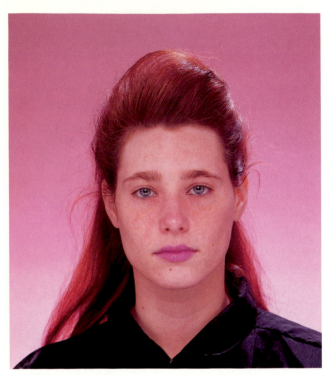

1 Before monochromatic hair-color application

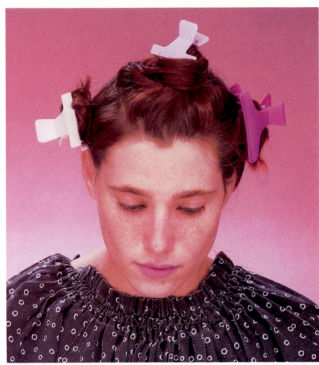

2a Divide the hair at the top section in preparation for color application and for ease of handling.

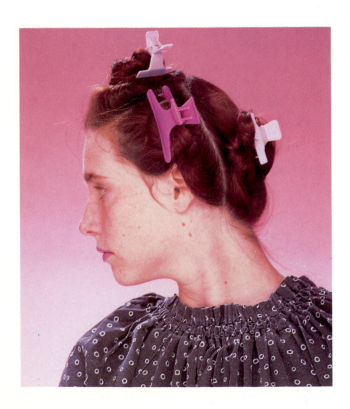

2b Divide the hair at the side section.

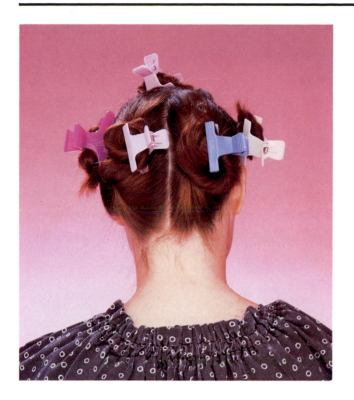

2c Divide the hair in the back section.

> Note: There is no set rule for applying monochromatic colors, but it is important to establish a routine for alternating colors. A pattern used for slicing is suggested — widen each slice considerably.

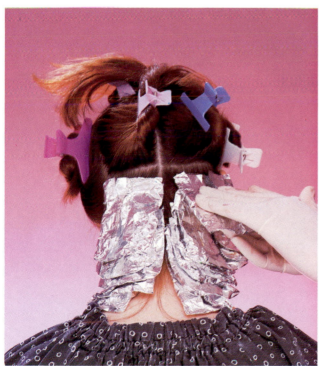

3 Starting in the back at the nape area, work toward the crown and completely across the head. Apply tint to horizontal panels until the back is complete.

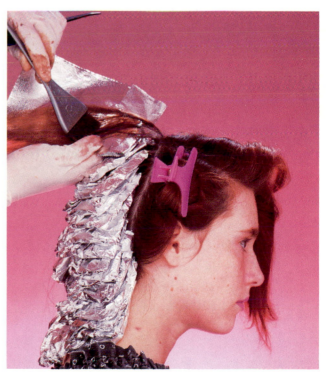

4 Start at the center crown and work toward the face frame. Apply alternating formulas to a wide center panel.

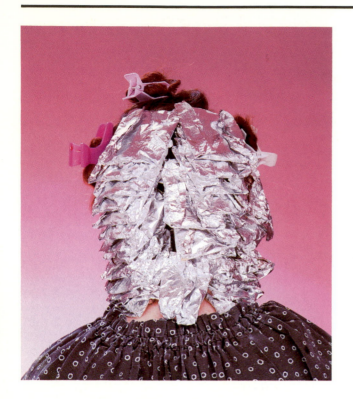

5 When the back is complete, continue the alternating procedure on each side and around the face frame.

Note: Because the hairline is inclined to absorb the color more readily than the hair in other areas, use a color level closest to the natural hair color, and apply it last.

6 Allow the color to process for 25-40 minutes (or follow manufacturer's instructions).

Rinse the hair thoroughly, and use a mild color-safe shampoo to wash the hair and scalp. Rinse well and use a protein conditioner or conditioning rinse if necessary.

The hair is ready for styling. See finished styles (montage).

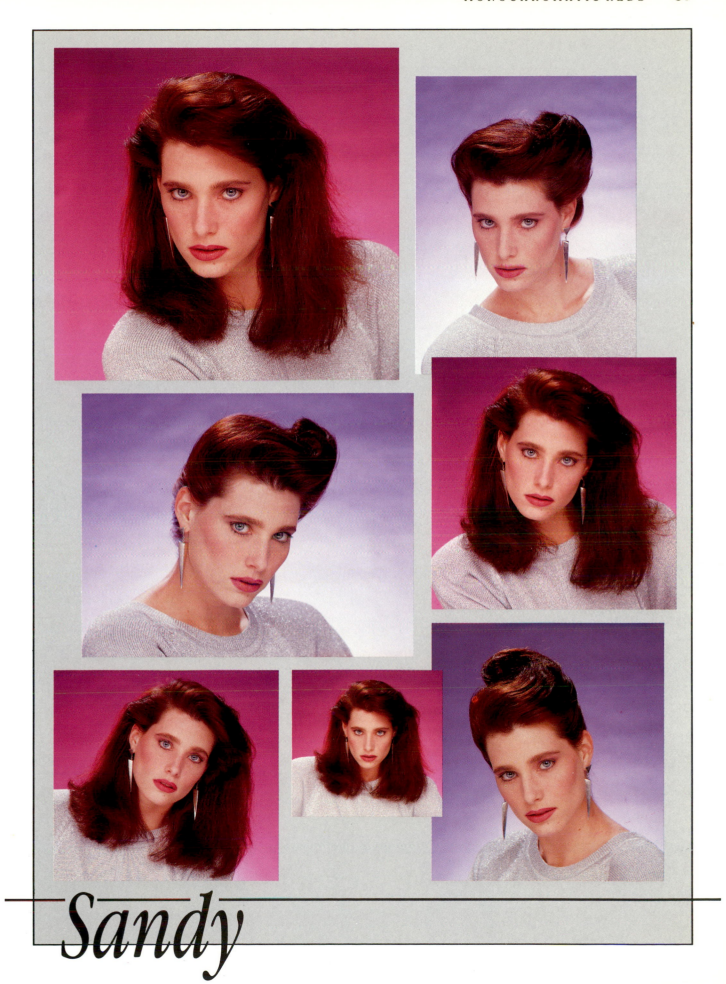

Sandy

Semi-Permanent Color

COVER AND SHINE FOR PREMATURE GRAY

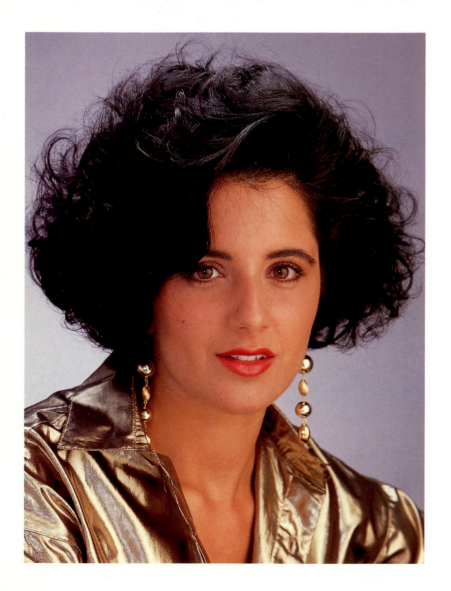

Premature graying from loss of natural color pigment occurs in clients of all ages, and both men and women can lose enough natural color pigments to demand attention.

This is a prime example of a young client who wants her gray hairs to be covered without undergoing a chemical tint. The obvious answer is a semi-permanent color product that will fade after a few shampoos.

No. **15** *Jeanine*

ESSENTIALS

COLOR FACTS

Most semi-permanent products provide non-oxidative color that has no lifting action so will not decolorize natural pigment. While it will not cover gray 100 percent, it will do a great job of toning and blending gray so it is not a glaring problem.

Semi-permanent colors usually contain conditioning properties, but their true value is that they stain and seal the cuticle layer of the hair and impart tremendous shine. A word of caution: When applying dark colors to gray hair, add a touch of red to the formula so the gray will not take on a greenish or ashen tone.

Note: Advise your client that the color will last through 6-8 shampoos — *not* 6-8 weeks, a common misconception.

HAIR ANALYSIS

Original hair color — Level 2, with approximately 10 percent gray showing at the temple and forehead areas.

DESIRED COLOR

A beautiful blue-black base with a healthy shine. If not completely covered, the gray should be camouflaged to a natural blend.

Tonal value — cool

Texture — excess curl, damaged by chemical relaxer

FORMULA

1 oz. rich cinnamon red — Level 7

1 oz. reddish bronze — Level 5

Note: Mix each color formula with developer according to manufacturer's instructions.

PROCEDURE

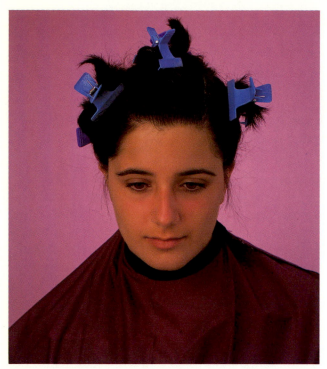

1a Divide the hair into easy-to-handle sections.

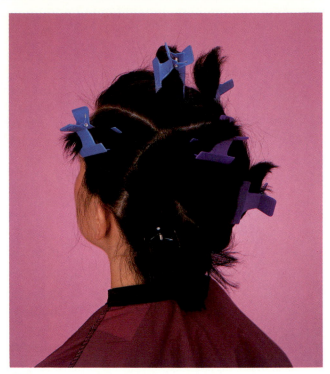

1b Easy-to-handle sections in the back

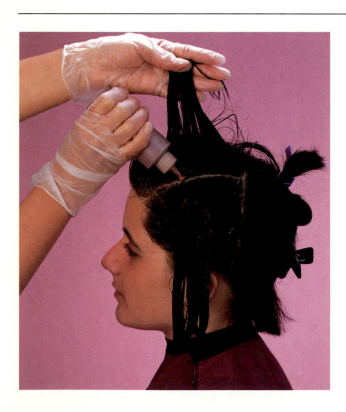

2 Mix formula ingredients in an applicator bottle and begin application where the style part will appear — in this case, in line with the left eyebrow.

Note: This is where gray hairs may be most obvious. By starting the application here, the product will have more time to process in that area.

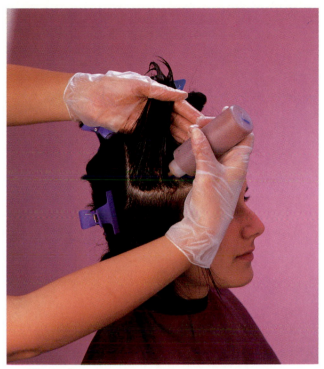

3 Work from the starting point at the crown toward the hairline on both sides, front and back.

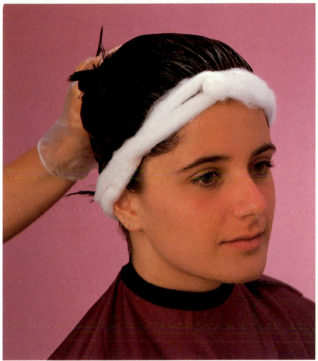

4 Place a clean strip of cotton around the hairline. Keep the cotton off the hair as much as possible so it will not absorb any of the color product.

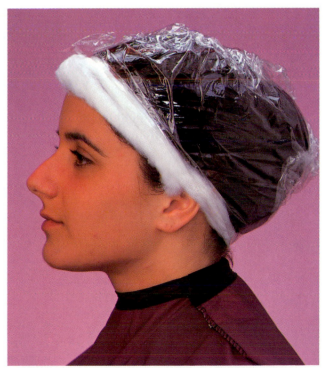

5 Cover the hair with a plastic cap and process under a warm dryer for 30 minutes.

6 After rinsing, towel-dry the hair and style using a diffused hand-held dryer and a "scrunching" technique to maximize volume and define curls.

See finished styles (montage).

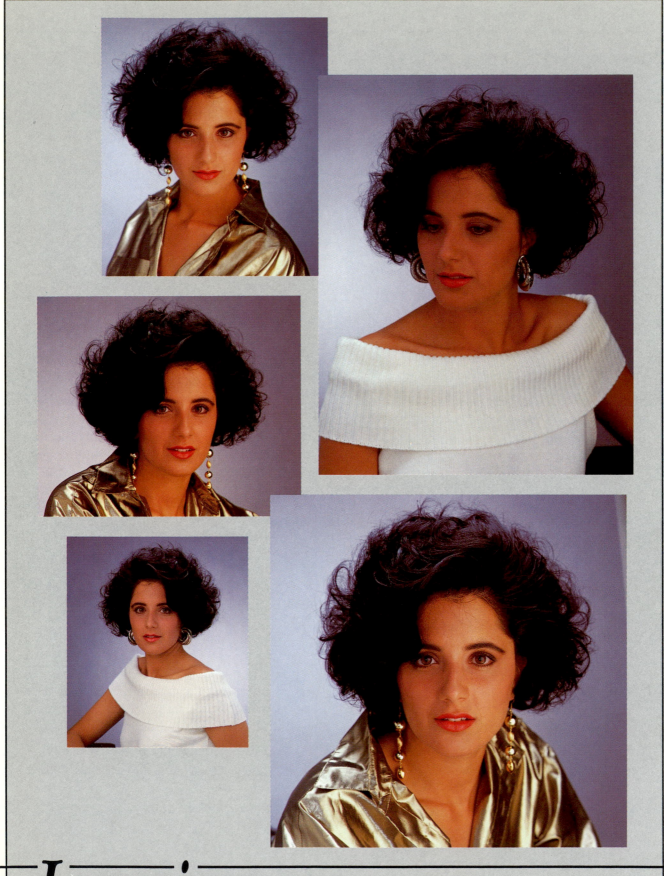

Jeanine

Blonde-on-Blonde Retouch

HIGHLIGHTING ON PRE-BLEACHED HAIR

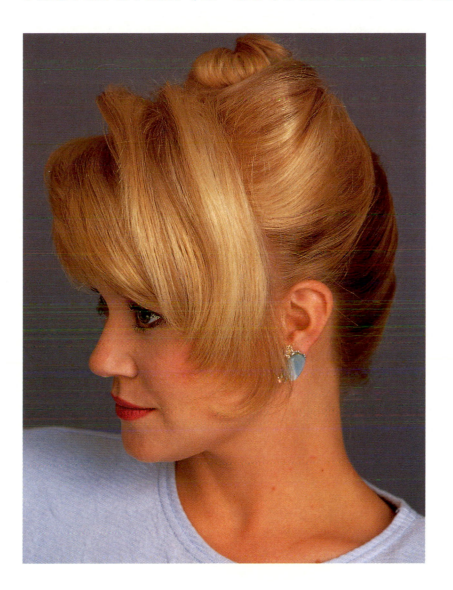

As a professional cosmetologist and color technician, one of your greatest challenges is to maintain a client's hair color, especially if it requires a highly stylized technique.

Almost anyone can change hair color initially without risking failure. But it takes a true professional to judge how to recapture the same color lights when the hair starts to grow out.

No. **16** *Jennifer*

ESSENTIALS

TECHNIQUE

The standard tint and two-process blonde touch-ups are relatively simple compared to refreshing highlights and lowlights in pre-bleached blonde hair.

This process is called monochromatic blonding, which you will recall means two or more levels of the same color with the same tonal value.

Often hair that looks beautiful after the initial high- or lowlighting process is destroyed in the retouch.

You will be challenged to new decisions: whether to increase the amount of blonde hair or maintain the same amount; whether to add darker strands to the hair, and whether to retouch only the new growth that has become too light.

The decision is yours and your client's. Your technical expertise will be called into full service. This illustrated maintenance retouch is a valuable lesson in color selection and technique.

COLOR FACTS

Whether you use several different compatible colors or several levels of the same color family, the colors must have the same tonal value — all warm or all cool. They cannot be mixed successfully.

Warm or cool hair-color products are usually identified on the package with a number followed by a letter or code that stands for either ash or gold tones. Manufacturers identify products differently, and as a professional you should get to know them.

HAIR ANALYSIS

Original hair color — approximate Level 7 (medium light blonde). The hair has been bleached to Level 10. The nape and lower back area was left natural, and highlights were added. Lowlights were added to the lightest blond areas. The hair colors have faded, and there is an outgrowth of 1–2 inches.

Tonal value — cool

Texture — smooth; lends itself to styles with minimum movement

Condition — very good, due to regular care

DESIRED COLOR

Pale, cool, iridescent blonde over most of the head, with darker, cool blonde lowlights. The portion of the hair left natural (Level 7) will have added cool highlights approximately three levels lighter than the base color.

SERVICE REQUIRED	Pre-bleach the new growth, then weave/foil highlights and lowlights throughout.
	Highlights: color lift
	Lowlights: color deposit
FORMULA 1	1 oz. creme bleach mixed with 2 oz. 30-volume (9%) peroxide (Level 10)
FORMULA 2	1 oz. medium blonde (ash) Level 7
	2 oz. 20-volume (6%) peroxide
FORMULA 3	1 oz. dark blonde (ash) Level 6
	2 oz. 20-volume (6%) peroxide

Note: Pre-bleach the new growth with Formula 1 — in the blonde area only — to Level 10 before you start to foil.

PROCEDURE

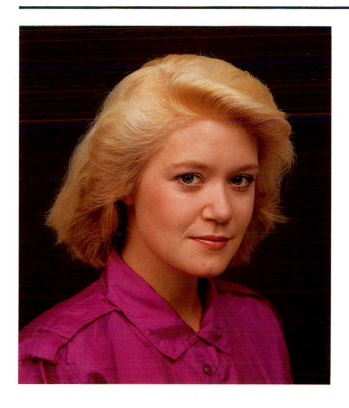

1 The hair as it looked before monochromatic retouch. The front is too light; the back too dark — almost no contrast in color from the original weave/foil is apparent.

Note: Because the color levels are faded to no apparent difference, this touch-up can be treated much as a virgin high- and lowlighting process. However, definite care must be taken to apply formula only to previously bleached strands.

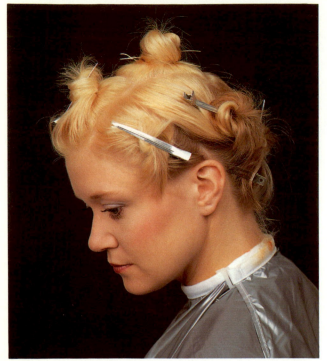

2a Divide the hair into panels no wider than can be easily handled and slightly narrower than the width of the pre-cut highlighting foil.

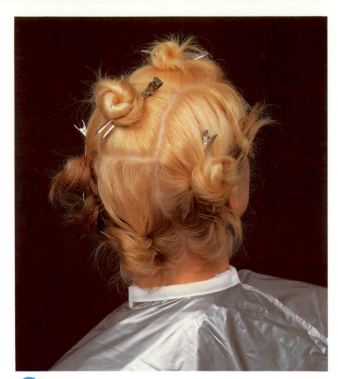

2b Divide the hair into panels in the back.

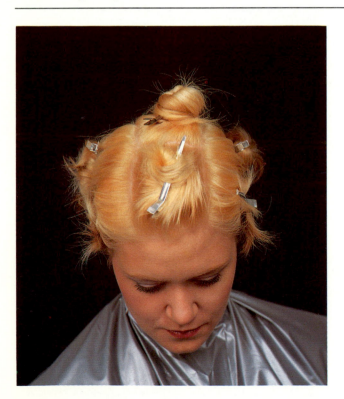

2c Divide the hair into panels on the top.

Note: Use pre-cut foil made of lightweight, non-slip material. It comes in a pop-up dispenser box for access to individual strips.

Mix both highlighting and lowlighting formulas at the same time.

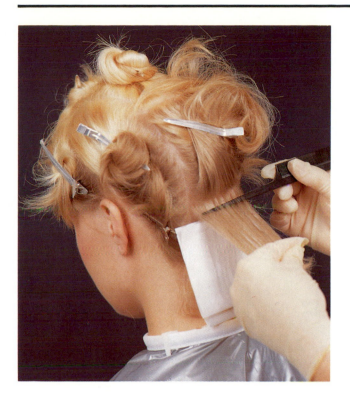

3 The darkest portion of the head will receive the lightest of the formulas (Formula 2). Start at mid-center back in the nape area. Slice and weave a narrow panel of hair.

Note: If a demarcation line is evident, indicating the outgrowth of the previous highlighting, you may want to apply bleach only down the strand to cover the new growth. This is your decision. This client's hair requires that the strands be lightened from scalp to ends to increase the amount of blonde.

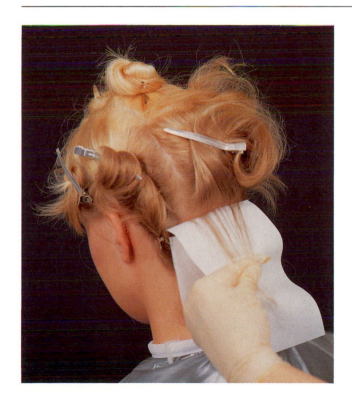

4 Slide the pre-cut foil strip over a tail comb and under the woven strands as close to the scalp as possible.

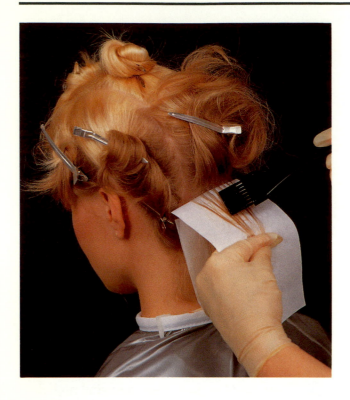

5 Apply Formula 2 to the entire strand. Turn the brush at an angle so bleach will only be applied to the darkest strands. Keep the application as light as possible, making sure the strands stay saturated.

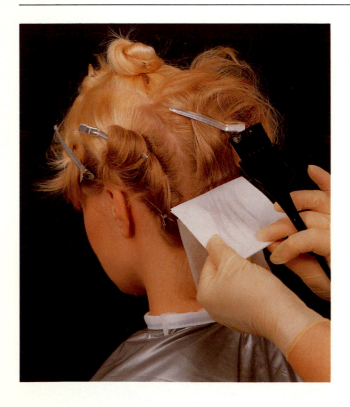

6 Because the foil strips are non-slip, it is not necessary to fold the sides. Only fold the strip once from end to the scalp. It stays in place without a clip.

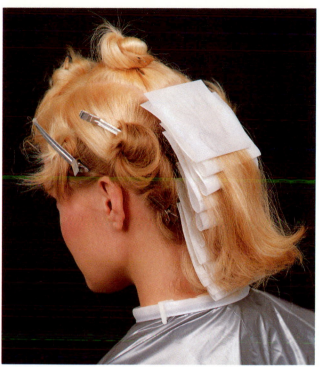

7 Skip a section ½ to 1-inch wide. Drop the hair not to be foiled and weave out the section directly above, using the same application technique.

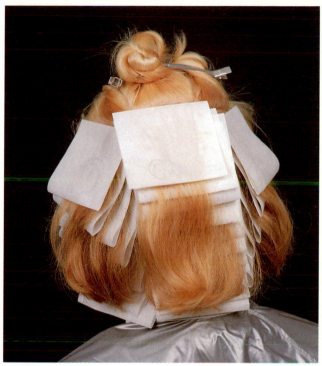

8 Complete the dark area requiring high-lift formula (Formula 2).

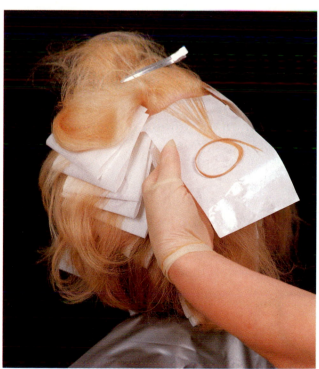

9 Starting at the crown, weave and apply the darker formula (Formula 3) to the lightest blonde area — crown, sides, and front.

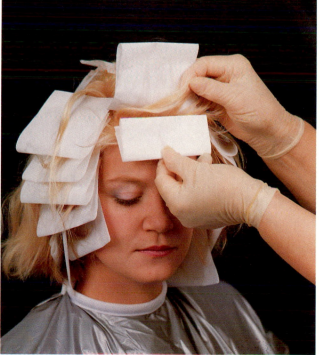

10 When foiling the hair at the front hairline, fold the foil strip twice to avoid covering the client's eyes.

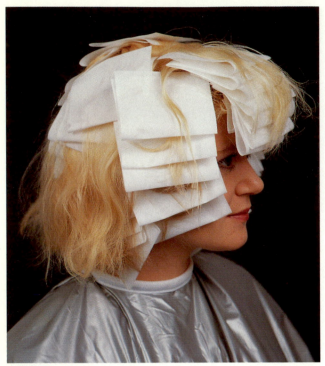

11a   All sections have been applied (side view).

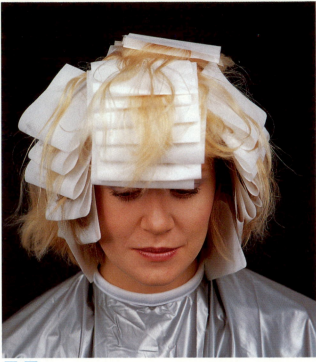

11b   All sections have been applied (front view).

12   During the processing, which can be 25–40 minutes, unfold foil strips in several areas to observe the degree of lift and/or deposit.

The results are rewarding — and you are sure to have a very satisfied client.

See finished styles (montage).

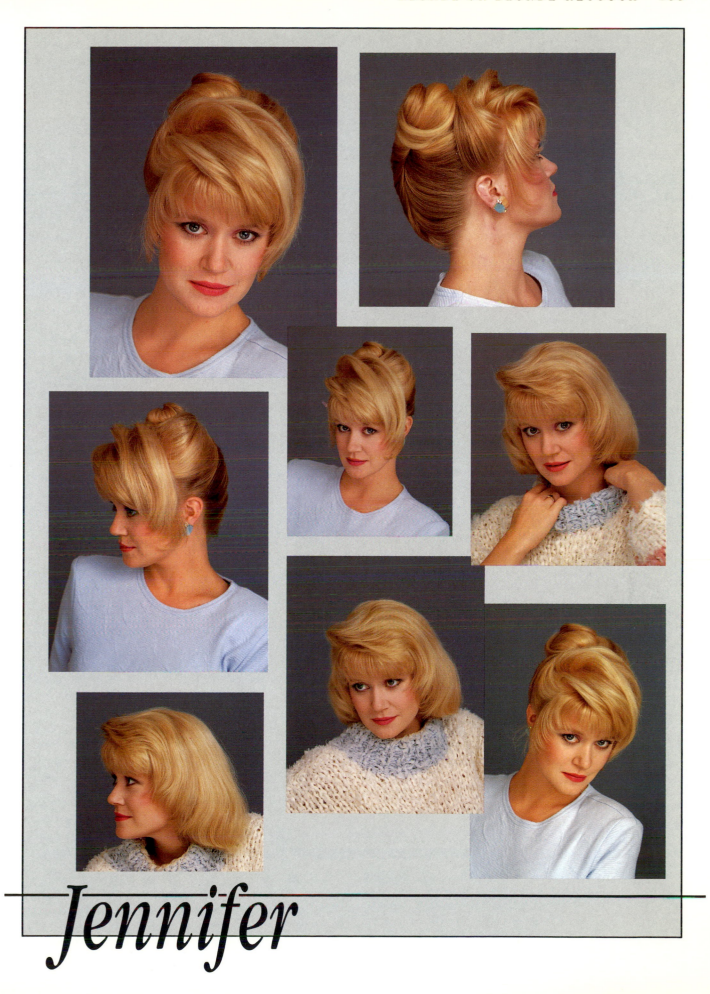

Jennifer

Surface Streaking

CREATING A HIGHLY ACTIVATED SURFACE SHINE

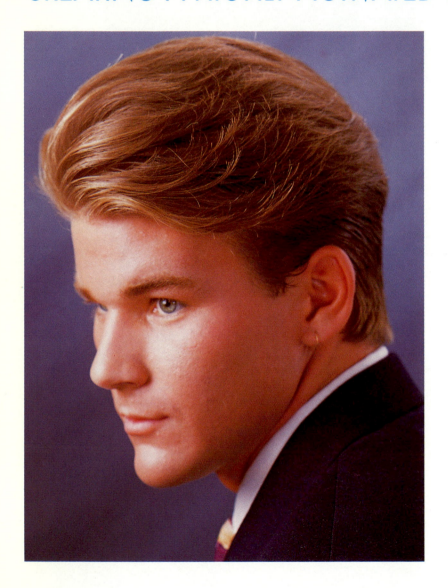

The ultimate hair-color service for busy men — those who just don't have time for personal pampering — must be fast, subtle, and easily executed.

Most men don't care for a salon service that is time-consuming or one that points out their vanity to other clients in the salon.

Surface streaking meets the requirements of speed and subtlety. You'll be surprised how quickly you can build a substantial male hair-color clientele if you cater just a bit to their instincts.

Men want to look their best. Personal appearance means a lot to them. They won't hesitate to work out in the gym or to have a chemical perm, but they are still shy about having their hair colored. Many believe the process is too time-consuming or messy. But it doesn't have to be either.

No. 17 Frank

ESSENTIALS

COLOR FACTS   The degree of lift and the processing time can be controlled by the volume of the developer with which you mix the powder bleach. Thirty-volume will lift color much faster than 20-volume. It is advisable, however, when applying powder bleach formula to hair color higher than Level 6, to use only 20-volume peroxide — and be prepared for about a 10-minute process. When adding highlights to a man's hair, it is recommended that you make the streaks no more than two levels lighter than the natural color. It will look as if the sun did it.

HAIR ANALYSIS   Original color — Level 6 with a few natural sun streaks

Tonal value — warm

Condition — excellent

DESIRED COLOR   The finished color should be the same warm Level 6 with natural-looking Level 8 highlights.

SERVICE REQUIRED   Surface streaking, using a comb-over technique

FORMULA   2 oz. 20-volume (6%) peroxide mixed with powder bleach to a medium-thick paste

PROCEDURE

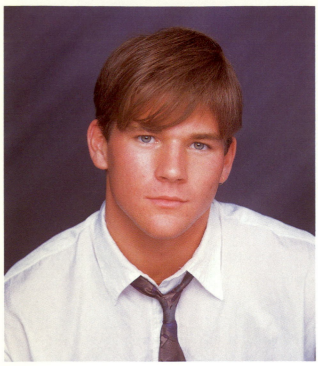

1 Before the surface streaking application, the hair was dull and uninteresting.

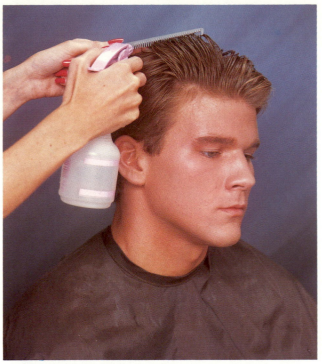

2 Wet the hair using a spray bottle.

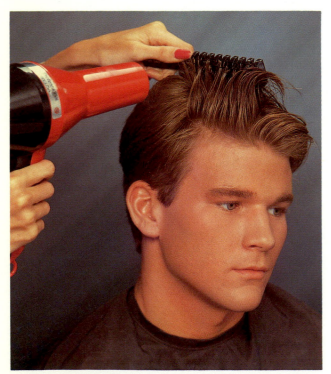

3 Style with a hand-held blow dryer.

Note: At this point mix the bleach so it will be fresh.

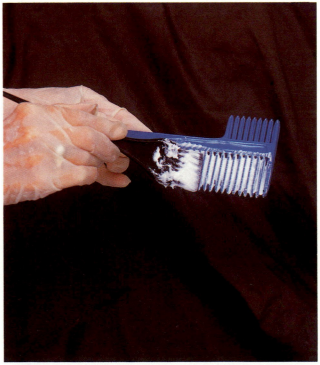

4 Brush bleach onto a wide-tooth tint comb (both sides).

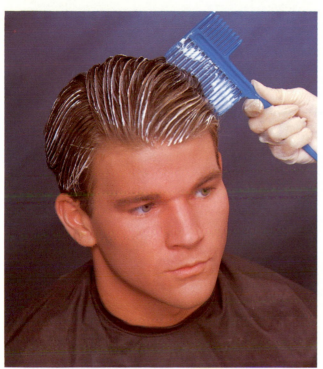

5 Starting at the front and using medium pressure, run the comb through the hair (front and crown).

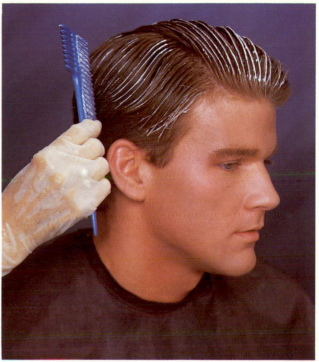

6 Reapply bleach to the comb, and comb through the sides and as far down the back as desired (usually only over the natural curve of the head).

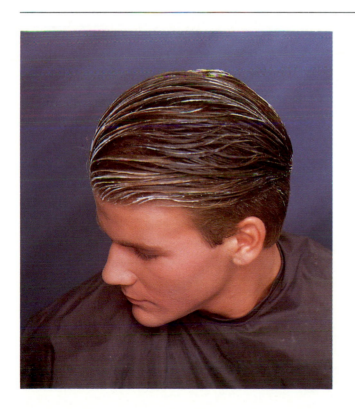

7 Allow the bleach to process for as long as it takes to lift the natural color to the desired level. Ten minutes is usually sufficient.

Shampoo the bleach from the hair and style as planned.

See finished styles (montage).

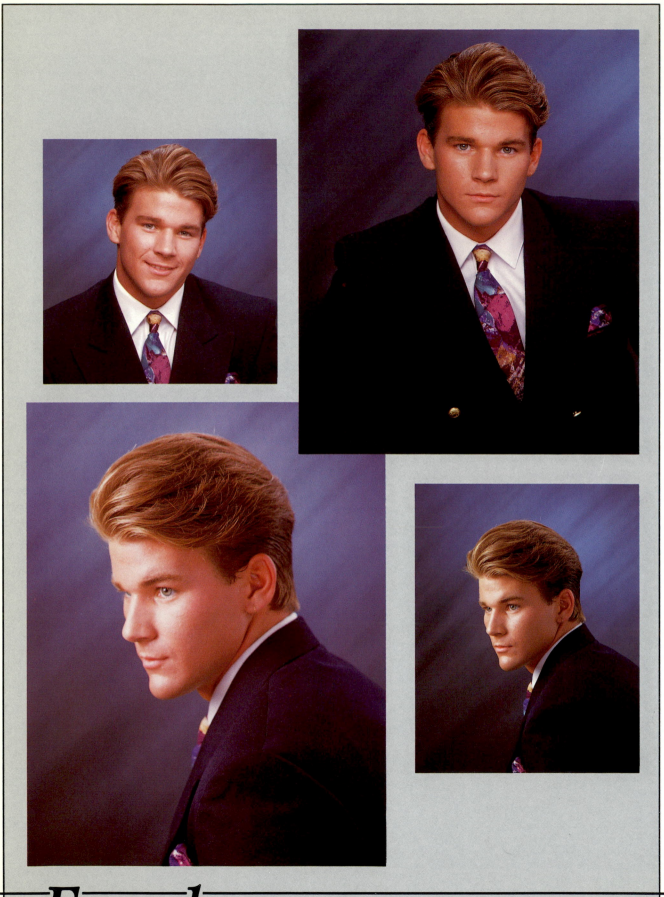

Frank

Glossary

HAIR COLORING TERMS

A

absorbent	able to take in and hold fluid
accent	in hair tinting, color used to highlight or emphasize color tone
activator	a chemical used in hair lightening or permanent wave solutions to assist in reaction
adaptability	in cosmetology, refers to harmony with head shape, face, neck, body features — also hair texture
alternating	occurring in reciprocal succession
alternation	multiple colors sequentially repeated
analysis	examining the hair to determine quality and condition
applicator	a small brush, stick, swab, or container used to apply a substance
art	skill in performance, as in art or painting
artificial	copy or imitation of something natural
ash	color with an absence of warm tones, also called drab

B

base area	the area nearest the scalp
brassy tone	the yellow, metallic appearance of poorly bleached hair
brighten	to make anything seem lighter or livelier, as in drab hair
bleach	a preparation to lighten hair by removing the pigmentation
blending	a process used to even color during retouches

C

color chart	a chart showing available hair colors
color filler	preparation for filling porous spots of hair during lightening, tinting, or permanent waving
color mixing	mixing of two shades for an in-between color

color rinse	a temporary color to highlight the hair
color wheel	a color-chromatic circle showing the correct positions of primary, secondary, and tertiary colors
complementary color	colors opposite each other on the color wheel that will neutralize each other
conditioner	a lotion containing acid or balsam
contrasting colors	two directly opposing colors
corrective coloring	process of rectifying undesirable color or tints
cosmetologist	a person trained and licensed to practice the art of cosmetology
coverage	the degree to which grey or white hair will take color
cream/creme	a mixture of two dissimilar substances whipped into an emulsion
cream lightener	thick substance under drabbing agent to neutralize unwanted red/gold highlights in the hair
cream rinse	product used to soften and add luster to the hair

D

decolorization	removal of color from hair
depth of color	describes degree of darkness or lightness
design	arrangement of shapes and lines to create a style with height and weight
density	the thickness of hair per square inch
development time	the time necessary to develop the desired color (also called processing time)
developer	a chemical oxidizing agent used in the process of coloring or bleaching hair
dimensional	the illusion of depth in a hair design
drab	a shade containing no red or gold tones

E

extra curly	hair texture (sometimes called "kinky") with tight, closed circle curls

F

face frame	the hairline surrounding the face
foiling	isolating, weaving, or slicing hair strands that are protected by foil strips during processing
formula	a combination of ingredients used to make a definite color

G

glazing	technique used to stain and gloss the hair's surface
graduated form	a hair design that graduates in length

H

hair color	products used to tint hair
hair density	number of hairs per square inch of scalp or body
hair lightener	chemical substance to remove natural color pigment from hair
hair	an outgrowth of the skin composed of keratin, a protein substance
hair tinting	adding color pigment to either tinted or virgin hair
high elevation	holding the hair at a 90-degree angle to the head while cutting
highlighting	bleaching or lightening selected strands of hair

I

icing	artistically adding subtle shine by using warm tones of non-oxidizing color products
intensity	the depth and brightness of color
indigo	a blue dye obtained from plants, used alone or with other vegetable dyes
ingredient	a substance needed as an element in a formula
isolated	kept apart from the mass

L

layer	a single horizontal thickness of hair separated from the mass
layered form	a design that features hair of various lengths throughout
level	the degree of lightness or darkness
lift	to lighten the color of hair only slightly, yet producing a definite change of color
lighten	to remove some color from hair
lighting-mixture	high-lift tint or bleach mixed with an oxidizing agent capable of removing color from the hair
line of demarcation	where natural hair stops and tinted hair begins
lowlighting	adding strands of dark hair color to lighter shades

M

mid-strand	portion of the hair strand between the base and the ends
monochromatic	multiple hair colors that have the same color base and tonal value but different color levels

N

neutralize	returning hair to a neutral state according to the pH scale, which measures acidity
neutralizer	an oxidizing substance that stops the chemical action of alkaline products
normal hair	hair that looks healthy, with no indication of damage or abuse

O

occipital bone	the base of the skull (forming the back of the scalp)
ounce (oz.)	a unit of measure of weight — $\frac{1}{16}$ of a pound
over-porous	the condition of hair that is excessively absorptive

P

parting	any line that separates portions of hair
peroxide	an oxidizing agent with a chemical code of H_2O_2
pigment	any color occurring naturally in the skin and hair (melanin)
porosity	the state of being porous
porous	containing tiny openings through which liquids can be absorbed
powder bleach	a fast-acting preparation containing sodium-perborate, hydrogen peroxide, and inert white materials
powder lightener	used primarily for frosting, foiling, highlighting (off-the-scalp) color services
pre-bleaching	a preliminary application of hydrogen peroxide or developer (various volumes) mixed with high-lift tint or bleach, applied to the hair to lighten beyond the level of the desired color
processing time	the length of time a chemical formula requires to be effective
progression	a succession of lines, shapes, or sizes that increase or decrease by proportional steps
protein	a class of complex amino acids present in all living tissue — used in quality hair conditioners

R

rat-tail comb	a comb with evenly shaped teeth and a tapered tail at one end
repetition	repeating or recurring in hair color — the same color used throughout a design
retouch	application of bleach, tint, or straightener to new growth of hair
regrowth	the new growth of hair after an on-the-scalp hair-color process

S

shade	degree of light and dark within a level
sheen	bright reflective light as seen on clean, healthy hair
semi-permanent	a color product applied to the hair without peroxide or developer; remains on the outside of the hair. Effects a percentage of gray coverage, and lasts through several shampoos
single-process	a coloring process that lifts and deposits color during the same application
stained	when color is not processed long enough to penetrate or oxidize completely; usually refers to a product made for use without an oxidizing agent
strand	a small portion of hair separated from the mass
strand area	the length of the hair, excluding an inch from the scalp and an inch from the ends
straight hair	hair with no curl, wave, or movement in the design
single application	product that lifts and deposits color all at once
solid form	a hair design that when viewed in shadow has a continuous form
slicing	extra-narrow panels of hair isolated for bleach or color application
surfacing	adding color or gloss only to the surface of the hair

T

tail comb	a thin comb with fine teeth along half of the length with a handle that tapers to a point
temporary color	a color rinse or toner product that imparts color or highlights and shampoos out
texture	the surface appearance or feel of hair
tonal value	the undertones present in all hair color, natural or synthetic, i.e., warm or cool
toning	addition of a color over pre-bleached hair

translucent	the property of a substance that allows light to pass
transparent	the property of a substance through which objects can be seen

V

virgin hair	hair that has never been tinted or bleached

W

warm	red and gold tones
wavy	a hair design that exhibits slow movement throughout
weaving	a technique of selecting minute strands of hair for highlighting by moving a tail comb in and out of a narrow panel